Plastic Techniques
in
Neurosurgery

Plastic Techniques in Neurosurgery

Edited by

James T. Goodrich, M.D., Ph.D.
Director, Pediatric Neurosurgery
Albert Einstein College of Medicine
Montefiore Medical Center
Bronx, New York

Kalmon D. Post, M.D., F.A.C.S.
Professor and Vice Chairman
Department of Neurological Surgery
Columbia University
College of Physicians and Surgeons
New York, New York

Ravelo V. Argamaso, M.D.
Professor of Plastic Surgery and Neurosurgery
Departments of Plastic and Reconstructive
Surgery and Neurological Surgery
Albert Einstein College of Medicine
Montefiore Medical Center
Bronx, New York

Foreword by Michael L. Lewin, M.D.

1991

Thieme Medical Publishers, Inc. NEW YORK
Georg Thieme Verlag STUTTGART · NEW YORK

Thieme Medical Publishers, Inc.
381 Park Avenue South
New York, New York 10016

PLASTIC TECHNIQUES IN NEUROSURGERY
James T. Goodrich
Kalmon D. Post
Ravelo V. Argamaso

Library of Congress Cataloging-in-Publication Data

Plastic techniques in neurosurgery / edited by James T. Goodrich,
    Kalmon D. Post, Ravelo V. Argamaso; foreword by Michael Lewin.
        p.   cm.
    Includes bibliographical references.
    Includes index.
    ISBN 0-86577-352-1.—ISBN 3-13-758801-4
        1. Brain—Surgery—Complications and sequelae.   2. Surgery,
    Plastic.   3. Skull—Surgery.   4. Facial bones—Surgery.
    I. Goodrich, James T.   II. Post, Kalmon D.   III. Argamaso, Ravelo V.
        [DNLM: 1. Neurosurgery—methods.   2. Surgery, Plastic.   WL 368
    P715]
    RD594.P53   1991
    617.4'80592—dc20
    DNLM/DLC
    for Library of Congress   90-11280
                                                                    CIP

Printed in the United States of America.

5   4   3   2   1

TMP ISBN 0-86577-352-1
GTV ISBN 3-13-758801-4

Pigmei gigantum humeris impositi plusquam ipsi gigantes vident

—Bernard of Chartres, 12th Century

To
Charles Dawe
Don Collins
Frank Visco
Tom Wert
John Lenanton
Robert Hoeppner
and the group at Orange Coast College, Costa Mesa, California

In June of 1968, a young, very tired, burnt out former Marine, just back from Vietnam, entered Orange Coast College to begin a career in pre-med. An extraordinary group of very talented and bright educational minds took an uneducated one and provided a never forgotten stimulus to become educated. To my giants at Orange Coast College, it is on your shoulders that I have stood. I have never forgotten your efforts and would like to thank you all now and dedicate my part of this work to you.

—James Tait Goodrich, M.D., Ph.D., FRCM (London)

To Linda, Illana, Alexander

—Kalmon D. Post, M.D.

To my wife Carol, and my children,
Sharleen, Susanne, and Stephanie

—Ravelo V. Argamaso, M.D.

CONTENTS

FOREWORD

Craniofacial surgery has moved from infancy to adulthood in less than a quarter of a century. Such a rapid development has been made possible by the close cooperation of the neurosurgeon and the plastic surgeon. Other disciplines, such as otolaryngology, dentistry, and anesthesiology, have made contributions to the field, but the neurosurgeon and the plastic surgeon have been the key players.

Surgery of the cranial vault in craniostenosis was practiced for over a hundred years, ever since Virchow defined its anatomic basis and Lannelungue performed the first craniectomy. However, reconstructive surgery of the cranium was a stepchild of neurosurgery. Only functional indications related to the central nervous system were viewed as justifications for surgical intervention. Existing or potential deformities of the craniofacial skeleton were ignored.

Maxillofacial surgery made vigorous strides since World War I, becoming ultimately an integral part of plastic surgery. Although the maxillofacial skeleton was part of and contiguous with the craniofacial skeleton, the plastic surgeon considered the orbit and cranium forbidden territory.

The collaboration of plastic surgeons and neurosurgeons was initiated by Tessier, Guiot, and their associates in the 1960s at Hospital Foch in Paris, and it became the model for craniofacial teams around the world. The subsequent spectacular progress in craniofacial surgery was based on a team approach. To be effective, members of the team had to understand each other's problems, had to be aware of each other's capabilities, and had to have some familiarity with each other's techniques. Everything had to be attuned to the social and psychologic consequences of severe deformities of the face and cranium, and prevention and correction of such deformities had to be a common goal.

The fruitful collaboration of the neurosurgeon and plastic surgeon was not limited to congenital deformities. It extended to the management of cranial trauma (a daily activity of most neurosurgeons) and to oncologic neurosurgery.

The introductory chapter of this book (Janecka) deals with basic biologic processes in wound healing and lays the foundation for all of the subsequent chapters.

Advances in plastic surgery have had a profound influence on the management of cranial trauma. In the chapter on cranioplasty, Hall and Goodrich present up-to-date choices of autogenous bone grafts and bone substitutes. Some of these choices, such as the cranial bone graft or hydroxyapetite, were not available two decades ago.

In the chapter on soft tissue repair (Goldstein and Strauch) the reader will find both classic plastic surgery procedures, such as contiguous flaps, and the more recently introduced microsurgical and myocutaneous flaps and tissue expanders. All of these procedures have an important application in the management of scalp defects or closure of spinal wounds.

In the repair of spinal myelomeningocele (Keating and Goodrich), a successful wound closure is of paramount importance. Neurosurgeons have often found themselves ill prepared to manage a huge soft tissue defect of the back and have called on their plastic surgery colleagues to collaborate with them. Recent advances in plastic surgery, such as tissue expanders and musculocutaneous flaps, are valuable contributions in managing these defects.

In the chapter on craniostenosis, Goodrich presents his own experience with current procedures for reshaping the cranial vault in congenital deformities. These are extensive operations consisting of mobilization and transposition of major segments of the cranial skeleton. The primary consideration is the correction of the craniofacial deformity. Advances in pediatric anesthesia and pre- and postoperative monitoring have made it possible to carry out these procedures safely, even in a neonate.

Many of these patients with Crouzon or Apert syndromes, hypertelorism, or orbital dystopia also have orbital and occlusal deformities. Their management is described by Argamaso in the chapter on facial disorders.

Thanks to the involvement of the neurosurgeon, the plastic surgeon is no longer confined to procedures on the mandible and maxilla: he can now include the orbit and the fronto-temporal area. The orbital cavity can be approached from all directions, including intracranially. The orbit can be osteotomized, enlarged, or translocated, and the ethmoids can be resected, while the brain remains protected.

The roof of the facial skeleton is the floor of the cranial cavity. This was formerly a no-man's land that neither the neurosurgeon nor the plastic surgeon dared approach. The plastic surgeon opened the way for his neurosurgeon colleagues to reach tumors in this region (Post and Blitzer). Plastic surgery techniques, such as mandibular osteotomies or musculocutaneous flaps, are essential in restoring the patient's appearance.

I congratulate the editors and authors for presenting their material in a succinct and readable manner through the combined atlas and text format. This book will not only be of value to neurosurgeons in managing skeletal and tegumental problems, it will be useful for all surgeons and their trainees in obtaining a rapid overview of what modern craniofacial surgery is about. The ultimate beneficiary will be the patient.

Michael L. Lewin, M.D.
Professor Emeritus
Plastic and Reconstructive Surgery
Albert Einstein College of Medicine, and
Former Chief
Combined Plastic Surgery Services
Montefiore Medical Center and Affiliated Hospitals

PREFACE

O! Author, with what words will describe
with such perfection the whole configuration,
*such as the sketch does here?**

O reader!, the same feeling which inspired Leonardo to restate the Vitruvian man and provide the perfect proportion inspired the editors to provide this palimpsestic atlas. The rapidly changing surgical techniques and the now-accepted, multiple surgical collaborations that occur in operating rooms both provided the stimulus for this book. In recent years wonderful collaborative efforts have developed between the various surgical services. One of the most useful has been the cooperation of plastic surgeons and neurosurgeons in the treatment of some of the more complex cases. The idea for this book came about when the three editors (two neurosurgeons and a plastic surgeon) realized the amount of useful information that was occuring as a result of the interface between neurosurgery and plastic surgery. The format is designed so that not only is the concept provided and discussed but the surgical technique is detailed step by step in an atlas format. The atlas-style format was selected in the belief that, like Leonardo da Vinci, neurosurgeons and plastic surgeons are more comfortable with the "visual" picture rather the written word—though both are provided!

This atlas starts with a discussion of wound management. No surgeon, in any field, can hope to design a good wound closure without an understanding of the principles of wound healing. Dr. Janecka has crafted a very practical presentation of wound closure and of the various types of suture material needed. The understanding of wound care and management is an important and very functional concept, and this chapter presents an excellent overview.

As neurosurgeons have attempted more complex surgical tumor resections and become more involved in facial trauma, the need for a better understanding of flap rotation and closures has become necessary. Drs. Goldstein and Strauch have reviewed the principles, along with the types of flaps that can be rotated or mobilized, for adequate closure. An understanding of these maxims will greatly enhance any neurosurgical practice.

The recent introduction of new materials and techniques has offered neurosurgeons and plastic surgeons a number of ways to correct skull or craniotomy defects. Drs. Hall and Goodrich have reviewed some of the classic skull-repair techniques and their pitfalls. The authors have also introduced some of the newer techniques using graft materials. This is a very practical chapter that all neurosurgeons and plastic surgeons will find useful.

Congenital malformations of the spine and calverium have long been a perplexing problem for neurosurgeons and plastic surgeons alike. In recent years the diagnosis and treatment of congenital malformations has changed in a number of ways. The authors review the techniques available for treating various congenital problems and offer helpful advice in managing the more complex anomalies.

Few neurosurgical procedures have undergone such dramatic changes as those seen in craniofacial reconstruction. The contributions of our plastic surgery colleagues have greatly influenced these changes. The chapter on Craniofacial Reconstruction examines the evolution of these innovations, from the days of doing just strip craniectomies to the full craniofacial reconstruc-

---

* Leonardo da Vinci, *Quaderni d'anatomia.* Christiania, Dybwad, 1911–16. Volume II, fol. 2r.

tions that are performed today. The principles behind the reconstruction and the various surgical techniques available are reviewed. The plastic surgeons have made a dramatic difference in how neurosurgeons will deal with craniosynostosis in the 1990s and beyond.

Plastic surgeons have made a number of important advances in the treatment of facial deformities. The work of Paul Tessier and others have provided many ideas and techniques for the correction of what used to be inoperable facial deformities. Many of the facial approaches require the complimentary skills of the neurosurgeon. Particularly in the area of facial trauma, the combined approach of neurosurgeons and plastic surgeons is now standard in most hospitals. Dr. Argamaso has outlined in chapter six the techniques available in working around the eyes, orbits, and midface region. Many of these techniques are now available to the neurosurgeon for facial reconstruction when working in collaboration with the plastic surgeon.

The treatment of tumors of the skull base and intracranial regions has benefitted greatly from the collaboration of neurosurgeons, plastic surgeons, head and neck surgeons, and maxillofacial surgeons. It can now safely be said that there are very few, if any, regions in the skull base and intracranial regions that cannot be approached, provided a surgical team concept is used. Drs. Post and Blitzer review many of the combined techniques available for operating in areas once considered neurosurgically inaccessible.

It is hoped that this book will further the collaboration between Neurosurgery and Plastic Surgery and allied fields, providing both the neurosurgeon and the plastic surgeon with many useful joint surgical ideas and techniques—all this for the improvement of patient care. Standards, techniques, and styles are changing so rapidly that, hopefully, this is a palimpsestic work, a work which will, in future editions, continue to add new techniques as they become available.

> *The knowledge which a man can use is the only real knowledge,*
> *the only knowledge which has life and growth in it*
> *and converts itself into practical power.*
> *The rest hangs like dust about the brain*
> *and dries like raindrops off the stones.**

James T. Goodrich, M.D., Ph.D.

---

* Harvey Cushing Laboratories. Then and Now, 1922, p. 9

ACKNOWLEDGMENTS

In infinito vacuo, ex fortuitâ atomorum collisione! The editors would like to thank a number of people, for through their fortuitous collisions, this atlas came about. When one realizes the efforts that are generated by so many people, in so many parts of the world, to make a book — yes, there needs to be many collaborations of minds and many did occur here!

We would like to start by thanking our editor, Hilary Evans, of Thieme Medical Publishers for her enthusiasm, gentle-but-firm prodding, and, finally, her constant encouragement to get this work out. What a great job you did Hilary! To Elyse Dubin, Kurt Andrews, and Kim Wright of Thieme Medical Publishers, Inc., what an extraordinary job your group did in getting the composition correct, the colors tightly hued, the infinitives unsplit—the end result a very handsome work and all to your credit.

To Helen Lopez and Esther Turull, for handling all the calls, mailing the bulky manuscripts, and reminding us to be nice and to be on time—thanks!

To Robert Demerest, our medical illustrator, thanks for doing such a wonderful job taking our obtuse operating room pictures and make them "visually readable" for the surgeon.

To our operating room nurses, such an essential part of any surgical team, for their watchful vigilance and their helpful advice and insight in preparing this manuscript. Hopefully this volume will also be helpful to operating room nurses elsewhere. To Terry, Mary, Annie, Carmen, Esther, Gloria, Katie, Vicky, Charisse, Audrey, Sandy, and Jean—a wonderful team to work with!

Finally, to all the authors for doing such a wonderful job in presenting some very complex subjects.

CONTRIBUTORS

Ravelo V. Argamaso, M.D.
Professor of Plastic Surgery and
  Neurosurgery
Departments of Plastic and Reconstructive
  Surgery and Neurological Surgery
Albert Einstein College of Medicine
Montefiore Medical Center
Bronx, New York 10467

Andrew Blitzer, M.D.
Professor of Clinical Otolaryngology
Director, Division of Head and Neck Surgery
Columbia University College of Physicians
  & Surgeons
New York, New York 10032

Robert D. Goldstein, M.D.
Associate Professor, Department of Plastic
  and Reconstructive Surgery
Albert Einstein College of Medicine, and
  Director of Plastic Surgery
Montefiore Medical Center
Weiler Division
Bronx, New York 10467

James T. Goodrich, M.D., Ph.D.
Director, Division of Pediatric Neurosurgery
Albert Einstein College of Medicine
Montefiore Medical Center
Bronx, New York 10467

Craig D. Hall, M.D.
Associate Director, Center for Craniofacial
  Deformities
Albert Einstein College of Medicine

Montefiore Medical Center
Bronx, New York 10467

Ivo P. Janecka, M.D., F.A.C.S.
Associate Professor
Department of Otolaryngology
University of Pittsburgh School of Medicine
Co-Director, Center for Cranial Base Surgery
Chief, Division of Head & Neck Plastic
  Surgery
Eye and Ear Institute
203 Lothrop Street
Pittsburgh, Pennsylvania 15213

Robert F. Keating, M.D.
Department of Neurosurgery
Director, Pediatric Neurosurgery
Oakland Naval Hospital
Oakland, California 94618

Kalmon D. Post, M.D.
Professor and Vice Chairman
Department of Neurological Surgery
Columbia University College of Physicians
  & Surgeons
New York, New York 10032

Berish Strauch, M.D.
Professor and Chairman
Department of Plastic and Reconstructive
  Surgery
Albert Einstein College of Medicine and
  Montefiore Medical Center
Bronx, New York 10467

Plastic Techniques
in
Neurosurgery

ONE

IVO P. JANECKA, M.D., F.A.C.S.

Principles of Wound Healing

The integrity of the human body is constantly maintained by a reparative and regenerative process called healing. Without it, life is not sustainable in any practical and durable form. It is essential that surgeons work in harmony with this natural phenomenon so as to enhance this healing process in the most favorable fashion.

The principles of wound healing are basically the same for all tissues and sites but do vary in terms of degree, duration, and the quality of healing at various regions. It is a well-known fact that the more complex the tissue, the poorer is its process of regeneration. At the present time, sophisticated organs do not regenerate but heal only with inferior tissue substitution. Even the organ of skin, for example, does not regenerate to its original form following injury, but only heals with a poor substitution known as a scar. This is explained on the basis of cell composition and the enormous energy and substrate needs for the process of repair. Simple cells can be totally utilized for the healing process. On the contrary, complex cells, normally engaged in their own specific function (e.g., endocrine and electrochemical) have their cell bodies devoted to that function with little "room" for basic reparative needs. A dedifferentiation of some ad-

vanced cells also occurs, permitting wound healing, albeit on a lower functional level.

Interruption of tissue integrity initiates a long sequence of events grouped under the term "wound healing." It is a complex process taking place on cellular, vascular, as well as systemic metabolic levels. The allowance of uninhibited progress of the healing stages to proceed is of paramount concern to all surgeons, but especially to those operating in critical areas. This chapter will attempt to provide an overview of wound healing with special focus on neurosurgical considerations. The encounter of critical structures during surgery, and the presence of various soft and bony tissues often bathed in the cerebrospinal fluid (CSF), creates special demands on primary healing. There is almost no tolerance to healing by secondary intention. The full awareness of the patient's general medical status and quality of regional tissues permits the healing process to be completed in a satisfactory fashion. The general medical considerations must include knowledge of any metabolic abnormality, since it is known that certain diseases, such as diabetes mellitus, may have a significant influence on the healing process. Also, results of previous therapies—local or systemic

1

—must be taken into consideration (e.g., previous scars and radiotherapy).

Our own surgical procedure must be harmonious with the regional blood supply, which is critical to the subsequent healing. Any tissue trauma creates an oxygen gradient between a hypoxic wound center and the wound periphery. This is desirable at a certain ratio, for it is one of the most important signals to vascular ingrowth. However, compromising tissue perfusion through unfavorable incision placement, tissue compression/destruction, or regional hypovolemia prevents primary healing with all its consequences.

Stages in Wound Healing

There are several basic steps involved in wound healing and they follow a progressive sequence (Table 1–1):

- Stage I: Inflammatory
- Stage II: Fibroblastic proliferation
- Stage III: Angiogenesis
- Stage IV: Connective tissue synthesis
- Stage V: Epithelization
- Stage VI: Maturation

Stage I: Inflammation

The purpose of this phase is the protection of the body from foreign substances as well as the elimination of devitalized tissues. There are two separate tissue responses during this phase: vascular and cellular. They are observed as changes in vascular permeability and movement of leukocytes into the wound.

Injury causes cell destruction, wound contamination, and vessel interruption leading to hemorrhage. The formed fibrin provides a scaffolding for subsequent migration of fibroblasts. However, a large amount of fibrin (e.g., a hematoma) inhibits migration of fibroblasts and endothelial cells, delaying the onset of stages II and III of primary healing.

The vascular response follows a sequence of initial vasoconstriction with vessel thrombosis for control of hemorrhage. This usually takes place within several minutes. Following that, there is a subsequent vasodilatation with leak-

age of plasmalike fluid from veins into the tissue. This is usually secondary to histamine, serotonin (from mast cells), and prostaglandins released in the wound during injury as well as the effect of proteolytic enzymes from granulocytes and macrophages. This causes the vessel endothelium (primarily the venous side of the capillary loop) to leak fluid into the interstitial space, possibly from an endothelial separation. Vasodilatation is an important step to subsequent phases of wound healing. The next stage of the blood vessel response following injury is the adherence of platelets, erythrocytes, and leukocytes to the vessel endothelium at the wound margins. This is followed by formation of fibrin and clotting of the lymphatics in the periphery of the wound localizing the inflammatory reaction by decreasing the drainage from the site of injury.

The cellular response of this inflammatory phase of wound healing (Tables 1–1 and 1–2) takes place from the 12th to 24th hour following injury and primarily centers on the activity of polymorphonuclear cells. They migrate out of the vessels into the tissue and become a part of the exudate. Also, macrophages are active and they represent the primary cellular element of this phase of wound healing. Their function is to remove debris as well as to attract fibroblasts to the wound. They become activated by breakdown products of fibrin. In the central space of the wound, tissue hypoxia increases the release of growth factor from the macrophages. This function ceases when tissue oxygen reaches normal level.

On the biochemical side, the prostaglandins are considered the mediators of inflammation. Specifically, prostaglandin (PGE_1) antagonizes vasoconstriction and PGE_2 attracts leukocytes. They can, however, be affected by aspirin and indomethacin, which inhibit prostaglandin synthesis. This may explain their principal effect as anti-inflammatory drugs. These prostaglandins affect the adenyl cyclase enzyme (responsible for synthesis of cyclic adenosine monophosphate), which mediates the action of serotonin and histamine.

Tissue pH also plays an important role in this phase of wound healing. Granulocytes are sensitive to low pH. In the inflammatory phase, following vascular stasis, there is tissue anoxia

Table 1-1. Wound Healing

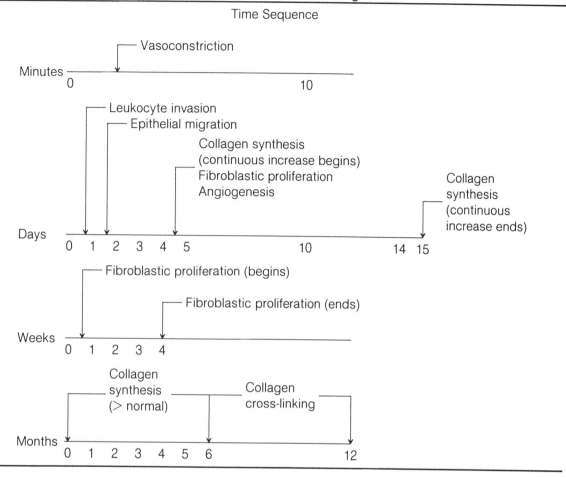

with increase of lactic acid accumulation (from glycolysis) and concomitant decrease in pH. This then causes lysis of granulocytes and subsequent release of numerous enzymes (including collagenase) with improvement of the solubility of local connective tissue.

Stage II: Fibroblastic Proliferation

This phase lasts from the first to the fourth week. Fibroblasts are the primary cellular components of this stage. They produce collagen, mucopolysaccharides, as well as collagenase when in contact with new epithelium. During the first 4 or 5 days, there is significant proliferation of fibroblasts as well as collagen deposition. It is of interest that fibroblasts do not recognize tissue specificity for the first 2 to 3 weeks. They originate mostly from blood vessel adventitia,

but may also come from undifferentiated mesenchymal cells. They migrate, proliferate, and produce glycoproteins and collagenase. They also activate latent collagenase. This is important in the eventual wound remodeling as well as in conditions of defective healing. One of the signals for fibroblastic proliferation is loss of contact with cells of a similar kind (effect of negative feedback mechanism). Also, macrophages and mononuclear cells activate fibroblasts, which produce a growth factor capable of suppressing the "growth inhibitory function" of pericytes (discussed later). Fibroblasts do not contain fibrinolytic enzymes.

Stage III: Angiogenesis

Angiogenesis begins from the fourth or fifth day and develops into what is clinically known, in secondary wounds, as granulation tissue. It be-

Table 1–2. Cellular Response to Wound Healing

Fibrin	Scaffolding for fibroblasts Breakdown products activate macrophages
Collagens	Secreted by fibroblasts Guides migrating epithelial cells
Fibroblasts	Originate in adventitia of blood vessels and mesenchymal cells Produce collagen, mucopolysaccharides, glycoproteins, collagenase Activate latent collagenase when in contact with new epithelium Attracted by macrophages Proliferate when contact with similar cells is lost When activated, produce growth factor that suppresses inhibitory function of pericytes Affected by oxygen level
Macrophages	Activated by breakdown products of fibrin Attracts and activates fibroblasts Produce proteolytic enzymes Release growth factor (induced by hypoxia) Immobilized by high level of zinc Remove debris
Granulocytes	Produce proteolytic enzymes (e.g., acid protease dissolving catgut) When lysed (by low pH), release collagenase Attracted by PGE_2 Sensitive to low pH Oxygen increases their phagocytosis Anti-inflammatory drugs diminish their action
Pericytes	Inhibit endothelial growth (during status quo) Fibroblast growth factor neutralizes the above function (during healing)
Epithelial cells	Migrate following loss of contact with like cells (negative feedback) Migration ceases following contact with like cells (contact inhibition) Replication is directly related to oxygen level Secrete collagenase
Angiogenesis	Begins as endothelial buds when suppressive effect of pericytes is neutralized by fibroblast growth factor Initiated by hypoxia Follow path of fibroblastic proliferation when fibroblasts activate latent collagenase

gins at the wound edge. Here, endothelial buds are formed, elongate and subsequently become new capillaries. They follow the path of fibroblastic proliferation. Hypoxia is an important stimulus for angiogenesis. The central space in the wound is hypoxic and thus creates a tissue-oxygen gradient. When this is eliminated, the new capillary growth also ceases. This phase of angiogenesis is essential to all components of wound healing and follows the activation of the "latent" collagenase by fibroblasts.

In a nonwounded tissue, the pericytes normally inhibit endothelial cell growth. When the effect of the pericyte on the endothelial cell is neutralized by fibroblast growth factor, released by activated fibroblasts, the endothelial budding begins with formation of new capillaries from the endothelial cells.

Stage IV: Connective Tissue Synthesis

Normal connective tissue is composed of collagen as well as elastin, the latter of which is not a replaceable component following injury and thus is absent in scar tissue. This stage begins on the fourth or fifth day with collagen synthesis.

Collagen represents 25% of total body protein and is considered to be a large glycoprotein (with a molecular weight of 270,000 daltons). It is secreted from fibroblasts in a monomeric form (protocollagen), which then aggregates through tropocollagen into fibers. Following its beginning on the fourth or fifth day, collagen deposition rapidly increases up to the 15th day post-wounding. This parallels the increase in wound tensile strength. Following that, there is no significant increase in collagen synthesis, but tensile strength of the wound does continue to increase, albeit with smaller increments. This is due to the inter- and intramolecular cross-linking of collagen. This takes from 6 months to 1 year to complete for skin and may be longer for other tissues. Eventually, only the functionally oriented fibers are preserved and all others are removed. This phase of connective tissue synthesis is characterized by the occurrence of embryonic collagen that eventually matures into the adult type.

Biochemically, collagen is characterized by: (1) three peptide chains; (2) glycine in the third position along the peptide chain; and (3) the presence of two amino acids (hydroxyproline and hydroxylysine, which are not found in other proteins). The original three peptide chains or protocollagen (helical coils bonded with hydrogen) form tropocollagen, and several tropocollagen units create filaments. They have parallel arrangement.

Stage V: Epithelization

The function of epithelium is to maintain internal homeostasis. The source of new epithelial cells following injury is the wound periphery or dermal appendages (hair follicles, sweat glands, and/or sebaceous glands) in partial-thickness wounds. These peripheral epithelial cells migrate over the wound bed and secrete or activate proteolytic enzymes (e.g., collagenase) that dissolve the overlying clot, permitting cell migration. This results in eventual separation of the eschar. The new epithelium, through the adhesive forces among its cells, gives this freshly epithelized wound its strength during the first 5 days. These cells do not have a strong attachment to the underlying tissue except, of course, in partial-thickness wounds. Therefore the new "scar" epithelium is very thin and fragile.

Following injury, there is an increase of mitoses in the basal layer of the skin with maximum increase in 42 to 72 hours. These cells subsequently migrate to the upper layers. The replication of these epithelial cells is directly proportional to the level of oxygen supplied. The signal for migration of epithelial cells is the interruption of their contact with cells of similar type, negative feedback mechanism. Migration, of course, ceases under normal circumstances when these cells come into contact again with other epithelial cells. This contact inhibition is not present between cells of different types. It is the collagen fiber that provides constant guidance to the migrating cells. The migration proceeds at the speed of several millimeters a day. It is of interest that, under normal conditions, mitoses have diurnal rhythm with greatest activity during rest. Following injury, this rhythm is eliminated and mitoses continue uninterrupted until the wound is healed.

Stage VI: Maturation

This end phase of wound healing encompasses collagen reorganization and wound contraction. During this phase, the haphazard orientation of collagen fibers is organized into a parallel pattern with significantly better mechanical properties. The least cross-linked collagen is removed in favor of a well-linked one and the fragile, soluble collagen is changed into a strong and insoluble one. However, in spite of significant increases in wound tensile strength even after 1 year, a scar is 15 to 20% weaker than normal skin. In an "old scar" there is still a dynamic balance between collagen synthesis and degradation. It is estimated that this metabolic process takes place within 5 cm around the wound. This phase completes the change of the embryonic type of collagen into the adult type.

Syndromes with Abnormal Healing

Lathyrism is a disease characterized by a loss of connective tissue structure, with subsequent/ skeletal deformities as well as aneurysm formation. It follows ingestion of seeds of *Lathyrus odoratus*, also known as sweet pea. The lathyrogen present is beta-amino propionitrile. In this condition there is no change in the quantity of tissue collagen, only in its solubility.

A similar lathyrogenic effect can be seen with the administration of penicillamine, which is a copper-chelating agent used for the treatment of Wilson's disease.

Ehlers-Danlos syndrome is a genetic defect of cross-linking of collagen. The deficiency is in the protocollagen peptidase. The protocollagen is not converted into tropocollagen. This is clinically manifested with hyperextensile skin and joints as well as tissue fragility and bleeding problems.

Marfan's syndrome is also a genetic defect of collagen cross-linking, especially manifested in the aorta.

Effects of Vitamins

Vitamin C is required for collagen synthesis in wounds and scars. It takes part in the hydroxylation of proline and lysine, which must be completed before they are incorporated into the peptide chain. Therefore vitamin C deficiency results in an incomplete collagen production affecting fresh wounds and old scars alike. Even in a mature scar, there is an active balance between collagen production and degradation. With vitamin C deficiency, an old scar becomes unstable and may even disintegrate. This reflects the resultant imbalance of the normal but continuous process of collagen degradation in a scar in the face of deficient collagen production.

Vitamin A is needed for collagen deposition. It is of interest that systemic administration of vitamin A reverses the negative effect of steroids and high doses of vitamin E on wound healing (discussed later). Topical administration of vitamin A increases epithelization retarded by systemic administration of steroids.

Vitamin E, in high doses, interferes with collagen production.

Effects of Steroids

Steroids affect wound healing in its early phase through inhibition of epidermal regeneration, fibroblastic proliferation, and suppression of capillary proliferation. Also, the later phases of wound healing are influenced by steroids through retardation of wound contraction. This occurs only following administration of excessive doses of steroids, not encountered in a clinical situation. However, even mild starvation, with resultant protein depletion (sometimes even induced by steroid anorexia), potentiates the effect of steroids on wound healing, so that even low doses of steroids may inhibit fibroplasia in such cases. Steroids have no direct effect on collagenase activity, but they do affect the cells producing collagenase.

Effects of Radiotherapy

Ionizing radiation affects dividing cells directly (by suppression of cellular proliferation) as well as tissue microcirculation through its effect on endothelium. It produces endarteritis with subsequent thrombosis and fibrosis. Of course, the observed effect of radiation is directly related to the dose and the rate of administration. It is possible to categorize the radiation effect into four phases. Phase I (first 6 months) is characterized by acute cellular damage. The second phase (second 6 months) is primarily reflective of the beginning of capillary fibrosis. The third phase (from 12 months to 5 years) signifies the progression of capillary fibrosis. In phase four (after 5 years) there is significant tissue fibrosis, atrophy, and possibly some necrosis. Also, radiation carcinogenesis may manifest itself in this phase.

Ionizing radiation does increase the risk of postoperative complications. Doses over 2000 rads create acute mitotic paralysis, which usually improves after 6 weeks. In higher doses, this risk lasts up to 2 years. It is thought that this is due to tissue hypoxia secondary to loss of small blood vessels. Eventually, radiated tissue may break down and result in radiation ulceration. This is frequently very painful and often reflective of much larger underlying tissue necrosis. The best treatment in such situations is meticulous local care, attempts to improve vascularity of the tissue by transferring a vascularized flap, as well as the possible use of hyperbaric oxygen.

Effects of Oxygen

Oxygen is an essential element of wound healing with a positive effect on phagocytosis of pathogens by leukocytes as well as proliferation and collagen production of fibroblasts. It also assists in development of new capillaries. Oxygen by itself can diffuse only a few microns from capillaries. It is of interest that a small degree of hypovolemia can significantly lower oxygen delivery to any injured tissue. Urine output and other measures of adequacy of systemic vascular volume and stability of perfusion of critical organs may be misleading in terms of adequacy of perfusion of a surgical wound. The connective tissue is quite vulnerable to vasoconstriction during episodes of systemic hypovolemia in which the body homeostatic mechanism is maintaining excellent perfusion of essential organs. This then makes the subcutaneous and connective tissues more susceptible to infection. Infected tissue also rapidly consumes oxygen, further worsening the hypoxia. An addition of 4 to 5 volume percent of oxygen to blood raises the arterial oxygen tension over 1000 to 1200 mm Hg (under hyperbaric conditions). This, then, increases tissue oxygen to a level sufficient enough to effectuate a bactericidal effect of cells. Increase in local tissue oxygen also not only stimulates collagen production, but also development of new capillaries. The effect of hyperoxia and antibiotics is additive.

Effects of Others

Anti-inflammatory drugs (aspirin, indomethacin) do not influence wound healing directly but through their action on prostaglandins. They also diminish granulocytic inflammatory action.

Cytotoxic drugs, in general, interfere with cell proliferation and thus affect the inflammatory phase of wound healing. Also, concomitant weight loss, frequently accompanying administration of cytotoxic drugs, causes nutritional impairment. This secondary effect results in wound healing interference (discussed later).

Zinc is needed in many enzymes. Significant trauma results in decreased blood and tissue levels of zinc. In patients who are zinc deficient, restoration of zinc levels to normal will result in an improved rate of epithelization, gain of wound strength, as well as an increase of collagen synthesis. Administration of zinc to patients with normal zinc levels shows no acceleration of healing. Excessive doses of zinc may result in immobilization of macrophages. Also, phagocytosis then ceases through the displacement of copper by zinc in some enzymes that are needed for collagen synthesis.

Anemia interferes with wound healing only when severe and if accompanied by hypovolemia. In such a case, the resultant capillary sludging and coagulation decreases oxygen delivery to the tissue. In general, wounds will heal in spite of severe anemia if blood volume is sufficient to maintain microcirculation.

Edema interferes with wound healing only in its severe form through mechanical and not biochemical influence.

Shock affects wound healing similarly to steroids.

Starvation, expressed in severe protein depletion, inhibits mitotic activity and adversely affects wound tensile strength. It is due to the lack of amino acid cystine necessary for collagen and mucopolysaccharide synthesis. If serum protein is below 2 mg per cent, inhibition of wound healing is observed with prolongation of the early phase of wound healing and prevention of the onset of the fibroblastic phase. It can be treated with lyophilized plasma. A high protein diet by itself does not shorten the early phases of wound healing overall, but does somehow shorten the rate of gain of tensile strength in the fibroblastic phase.

Complications of Wound Healing

Failure to achieve primary healing is considered a surgical complication. There are numerous factors that come into play and cause an alteration in the normal sequence of wound healing. They can be categorized into a systemic group as well as a local or regional category. The common denominator to the local or regional factors influencing wound healing is tissue hypoxia. The causes, of course, can be multifactorial, ranging from the effect of trauma, infection, malignancy, to the presence of a foreign body, radiation arteritis, coagulation necrosis of burns, among others. It is important that the surgeon's influence on the local factors prevents progression of tissue hypoxia to ischemia. It is safe to say that all ischemic wounds are hypoxic, but not all hypoxic wounds are ischemic. Ischemic wounds eventually end up with some degree of tissue necrosis, either on a microscopic or a macroscopic level.

The systemic group of factors influencing wound healing can be subcategorized into: (1) metabolic factors (e.g., diabetes mellitus, nutritional disorders); (2) circulatory factors, primarily due to tissue hypovolemia with decrease of tissue oxygen tension (PO_2), (e.g., severe anemia, peripheral vascular disorder, and vasculitis of various etiologies); (3) hormonal factors, which also encompass the administration of steroids; and (4) autoimmune factors, frequently encountered in patients with rheumatoid arthritis who have an increased amount of collagenase present, primarily in the synovial fluid. (This is usually manifested in a form of cartilage destruction of the affected joints.) Also, in these patients, the prolonged use of steroids further complicates the wound healing problem.

Surgical infection seems to be directly related to tissue hypoxia and often begins in poorly vascularized tissue. In general, poor tissue perfusion leads to the decrease of available oxygen at the cellular level, which affects the leukocyte phagocytic function. Poor perfusion also limits the delivery of immune substances to the wound as well as the removal of carbon dioxide. This, then, leads to further worsening of local perfusion with vessel thrombosis and possibly even tissue necrosis. It is safe to say that the overall wound resistance is related to tissue oxygenation. As previously stated, local tissue dehydration makes the wound more susceptible to infection due to its effect on tissue perfusion and oxygen saturation. The subcutaneous PO_2 is thus a more reliable indicator of a true volume resuscitation than, for example, urine output. Therefore the best prevention of infection is adequate tissue perfusion assuring oxygen delivery.

Acute surgical infection in a healthy patient is usually related to tissue viability or the presence of dead space. The design of surgical incisions, flap elevation, and reconstructive measures must take into account the normal vascular pattern of the surgical site or any previous interference with it (e.g., scars and radiotherapy). In general, an approach phase of any surgical procedure usually involves a transposition of uninvolved tissues (e.g., skin or muscle flaps) to permit visualization of involved structures. Tissue folding, under tension of stay retraction sutures and its significant desiccation with exposure to the operating room lights, is often sufficient to embarrass the local circulation. Finally, wound closure under tension, underlying hematoma, or tight dressing may be the critical factors resulting in tissue necrosis or infection.

Complications may be broadly placed into several groups, depending on where the error or "act of God" took place from the moment of surgical planning to the end of wound maturation.

1. *Complication in design* is a discrepancy between the theoretical plan and the final outcome of a surgical procedure. Modifications, on the basis of patient's age, general health, desires, as well as loco-regional tissue status, may have to be considered when selecting a surgical technique. Estimation of the procedure's predictable success, functional and aesthetic limits enter into the balancing equation between the original surgical concept and the achievement of its final purpose.

2. *Complication in execution* usually signifies a technical error. Correct preoperative markings, simply performed on an awake, sitting, or standing patient (even the day before), help with the precision of surgical planning. It also assures that the patient's positioning on the operating room table does not compromise the plan of the surgical exposure. Simplicity should be the guiding principle. Atraumatic surgical technique, a respect for tissue viability, and a true understanding of regional wound healing specifics, set the framework for primary healing. Elimination of wound dead space with a drain or tissue transfer is an important addition.

3. *Complication in healing biology* is primarily related to tissue hemodynamics, resulting in inadequate oxygen delivery and carbon dioxide removal. If, for example, skin perfusion drops below 1 to 2 cc/100 g/min for a prolonged period of time, tissue necrosis ensues. Biologic as well as physical factors play a significant role here. Time-tested clinical evidence of dermal bleeding or capillary refill is good evidence of adequacy of tissue blood supply at that moment, but it does not guarantee an uncomplicated

healing. Tissue perfusion is a dynamic process changing in real time. Our purpose as surgeons is to assist and not to interfere with this process of wound healing. There are some limited steps we can take to help with borderline perfusion of soft tissues. First, eliminate any potential external compression (e.g., tight dressing) or release wound tension (positioning, flap release, evacuation of hematoma, etc.). Second, some pharmacological agents do have a known beneficial effect on tissue circulation in special circumstances. For example, dextran (low molecular weight) lessens slugging of red blood cells in capillaries and dipyridamole as well as aspirin, through their effect on platelets, decrease the chances of intravascular clotting. This concomitantly improves the flow.

4. *Complication of endurance* signifies a mismatch of long-term wound demands on the method of repair. The tissues, for example, may not withstand external pressure, adjuvant therapy, internal implants, or contain patient's own CSF fluid. A potential susceptibility of tissue to infection (e.g., overlying acrylic cranioplasty) or cancer (previously radiated or burned tissue) deserves our consideration in the planning stage to avoid the ultimate reversal of the surgical procedure.

How to Optimize Primary Healing

It is every surgeon's plan to achieve primary healing of a surgical site with minimal functional and aesthetic consequences. The actual outcome is, however, sometimes significantly different and often understandable in retrospect. Familiarity with biologic principles of wound healing and all potential factors of interference with this process in a specific patient gives us a solid base to harmonize healing. The surgical axioms of "gentle" handling of tissue, "adequate" hemostasis, and "tension-free" closure are familiar to all surgeons. The practical application of these principles is what can be called "surgical experience." The judgment of how far to go, how much to remove, and where to get tissue substitution often makes the difference between satisfactory and unsatisfactory wound healing.

Since it is self-evident that primary healing is directly related to tissue viability, it is preferable to close all wounds at all levels with vascularized tissue. The successful use of autogenous, but nonvascularized tissue (e.g., grafts — bone, skin) depends on the vascularity of the recipient site as well as the adequacy of graft stabilization. Because new vessel ingrowth, within a limited period of time following transfer, is critical to graft revascularization and thus reintegration of it at a different site, it imposes significant demands on the wound to achieve primary healing.

Alloplastic materials serving as tissue substitution in special situations have a long and basically satisfactory track record in surgery. The fact that they do not become revascularized poses a permanent risk of infection. This handicap should be balanced against implant's potential for excellent contouring, relative ease of application, and limitless availability.

Wound closure should encompass most, if not all, layers invaded during surgery. This concept will automatically eliminate dead space often created with removal or transfer of tissue, which is a potential source of wound healing problems and should be dealt with prior to completion of closure. Even large potential space (e.g., a temporal fossa without temporalis muscle) can be easily coapted with a mobile overlying scalp. This is best assisted with a closed suction system, which accomplishes an immediate contact of the scalp with the depth of the defect (through negative pressure) and removes postoperatively any extravasated blood from this site. The use of drains should be individualized. They should not be placed directly over, for example, freshly repaired dura. It is possible, however, to use suction drains even in such cases if the drain is placed at a distance from the dural repair. The achieved direct and immediate contact of the scalp with the dura (secondary to some negative pressure) permits the wound healing to proceed from that moment on and not be interfered with by the presence of some hematoma when a drain is not used. It is unlikely that, when placement of a drain is performed in accordance with the wound demands, the drain itself would produce a CSF leak. It is more plausible that when a leak developed, it was there from the beginning, but masked for several days by the presence of a hematoma. CSF does possess hemolytic properties.

Table 1–3. Tensile Strength of Wound

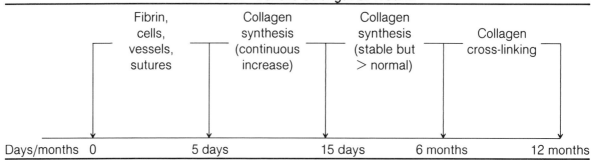

Fibrin, cells, vessels, sutures	Collagen synthesis (continuous increase)	Collagen synthesis (stable but > normal)	Collagen cross-linking	
Days/months 0	5 days	15 days	6 months	12 months

Principles of Wound Closure

Primary closure of a wound encompasses reapproximation of tissues interrupted by either trauma or elective surgery. It reflects the surgeon's recognition of the difference between a clean, contaminated, or infected wound. A clean wound can be routinely closed. A contaminated wound should be converted into a clean one before closure (e.g., debridement, removal of foreign bodies, irrigation, etc.). An infected wound should not be closed because the conversion into clean wound normally requires time-dependent treatment.

Primary closure reflects reestablishment of tissue continuity through approximation of various layers. This is most frequently accomplished with sutures.

Suture material should be selected to maintain edge-to-edge apposition of specific layers until collagen is synthesized and forms a permanent bond. Cells, blood vessels, ground substance, and fibrin contribute to the development of tensile strength in the first 2 to 5 days, and in some areas of the body sutures are removed at that time (Tables 1–2 and 1–3). Therefore a wound is held together in the first few days only by nonfibrous material. This makes wounds fragile.

Sutures and Suturing

Suturing of a wound accomplishes approximation of its layers and, for a limited period of time, maintains its tensile strength. The objective of using sutures is to add physical strength to an interrupted surface, obliterate a space, and stop capillary oozing. Each suture is expected to fulfill specific tasks.

The selection of a suture material depends on several basic requirements of the wound:

1. Closure of external or internal surface
2. Degree of wound tension
3. Extent of contamination

There are two distinct categories of suture materials: absorbable and nonabsorbable. They can be further subclassified into monofilament and multifilament, natural or synthetic fibers.

Absorbable sutures include catgut, which is derived from the submucosa of sheep intestines or the serosa of beef intestines. It is a relatively weak suture. If more resistance is required, it is treated with chromium, giving chromic catgut. Following placement in the wound, catgut is digested by acid protease, which is produced by inflammatory cells. This process is slightly slower in chrome-treated than in plain catgut. The rate of digestion, however, varies among individual sites. The plain catgut incites a greater inflammatory reaction than chromic catgut.

Collagen sutures are prepared from long flexor tendons of steer. They are usually made for ophthalmic surgery.

Polyglycolic acid and its copolymer (polyglactin 910) are prepared from monomers. They do not depend on the enzymatic reaction for absorption and are slowly hydrolyzed by water. The disappearance of these sutures takes place in about 80 days for the polyglactin 910; it is about 100 to 120 days for the polyglycolic acid. Both catgut and the synthetic absorbable sutures lose their strength more rapidly than they disappear from the wound. In general, catgut has lost about 50% of its strength in 20 to 30 days as well as the polyglactin 910. Polyglycolic acid loses strength even faster.

Nonabsorbable sutures include silk, cotton, nylon, polyester (Dacron), polypropylene, and steel. Nylon and steel exist in both monofilament and multifilament form. Silk is classified as a nonabsorbable material, but it does gradually lose its tensile strength and after about 1 year it has no strength at all. It usually disappears from the wound in 2 years. Nylon will swell in the tissue and lose about 20% of its initial strength after 1 year.

Some sutures are coated with silicone oil to prevent abrasion during the passage through the skin and some polyester sutures have been impregnated with Teflon. However, the coating materials often detach from the suture and are deposited in the wound. Small granulomatous reaction may develop. All nonabsorbable sutures induce cellular reaction. Silk and cotton produce the greatest reaction, followed by polyester and nylon. Polypropylene and steel are the least reactive suture materials. In an uninfected wound, the cellular reaction is microscopic and seldom involves an area greater than twice the diameter of the suture.

The reactivity of a suture is important in areas close to the body surface. In the presence of bacterial contamination or infection, catgut will be absorbed more rapidly. This is because of the presence of a large number of inflammatory cells, which increase the concentration of the proteolytic enzymes normally dissolving catgut. Synthetic absorbable sutures are not affected by inflammation, but all sutures function as foreign bodies causing prolongation of existing infection. Multifilament sutures can be penetrated by bacteria but not by the inflammatory cells. This permits sequestration of bacteria within the sutures. Monofilament sutures do not provide this environment for bacteria.

Handling qualities of sutures must also be considered by surgeons. Multifilament sutures are easier to handle than monofilament sutures. They lie flatter on the wound but may be more difficult to remove. Also, synthetic sutures require more surgical knots during tying than natural fibers because the synthetic fibers possess "memory," attempting to return to their original (straight) configuration. Synthetic absorbable sutures handle like silk, which has the best handling qualities of all sutures.

Selection of sutures should respect the biologic properties of the wound and mechanical specifics of the suture. The rate of healing and suture disintegration must also be considered.

It is important to realize that sutures are not needed after the wound has healed. Retention of skin sutures permits epithelial migration along the sutures with formation of suture tracts. In tissues with a prolonged healing sequence, e.g., fascia (its ultimate strength is not attained for almost a year), it is suggested that such layers be closed with nonabsorbable materials.

Suturing

Placement of a suture in a specific layer or plane is fundamental to good surgical technique. Sutures, expected to provide temporary wound strength (collagen fibers cannot be recognized in human wounds before the seventh to ninth day), should be placed in fibrous structures (e.g., dermis) and removed after 5 to 10 days in order to minimize the potential for stitch abscesses and suture marks. Subcuticular sutures eliminate this potential problem.

Soft and nonabsorbable materials are preferably used. External epithelium of a wound can be further adjusted with a fine suture or tape. For this purpose, nonabsorbable material or chromic catgut are selected to keep the surface skin reaction to a minimum.

Delayed Primary Closure

Delayed primary closure refers to wound approximation several days after the wounding incident (trauma, surgery). Several reasons exist for selection of this option: the uncertainty of tissue viability, high infection potential, as well as inadequacy of volume for soft tissue closure without tension. This delayed closure method can be selected only in noncritical areas. For example, an underlying dural repair, bone grafts, etc., would not be suitable for this method. In such situations, tissue viability and size adequacy must be determined intraoperatively and tissue substitution methods (e.g., flaps) are selected. In traumatic wounds, the tissue infection potential is balanced by wide debridement, proper drainage, intravenous antibiotics, and a predictable vascularized flap transfer.

Closure of Secondary Wounds

Closure of secondary wounds (e.g., exposed craniotomy, CSF leak) requires specific analysis of factors that contributed to the formation of a secondary wound. Tissue blood supply, surgical technique used, and infection may have all played a role. The wound must be considered "stable" prior to any attempt at closure. That means "reading" of the wound by the surgeon, identifying an absence of an acute infection, demarcation of tissue necrosis, and judging the patient's overall stability. The closure should be accomplished with the simplest, but the most predictable, method (e.g., arterialized vs. random flap).

Principles of Wound Care

Surgical care of any wound must be in harmony with the local, regional, and systemic factors. Wound care cannot be looked on as an isolated, local event. Diagnostic evaluation usually focuses on the clinical assessment of the wound and the surrounding region (e.g., vascularity and signs of infection). In rare instances, an x-ray evaluation (for foreign body) is useful. Wound culture may be useful as a guide to the offending organism if an infection subsequently develops. However, there is not a direct correlation between a result of culture from a contaminated wound and the pathogen of a subsequent infection.

Care of a surgical wound actually begins before the knife engages the tissues. The preparation and shaving of the surgical site should be done immediately prior to surgery. Shaving should not be done the night before because it creates minor abrasions with contamination, resulting in the onset of an inflammatory phase before surgery. It is helpful, however, to use a simple wash (e.g., pHisoHex) of the surgical site the night before surgery. For craniotomies, this may incorporate shampoo of the hair, which is probably equivalent in its cleansing efficacy to the actual "full shave" prior to surgery. The main advantage of extensive shaving is in simplicity of manipulation of the surgical area now devoid of sometimes long and cumbersome hair.

In general, a surgical site should not come into contact with potentially harmful liquids (e.g., full-strength peroxide, iodine, or Dakin's solution). Skin preparation is best done with standard solutions (povidone iodine, pHisoHex, etc.) remembering the gravity effect on any preparative solution with a potential pooling of it in a dependent area for the duration of surgery. Skin coverage with, for example, a transparent sheet of plastic (Steri-drape) appears to increase the "protection" of the surgical region. However, from the practical point of view, once an incision is made, the previously adherent plastic begins to separate, providing space for fluid accumulation during surgery, eliminating any real advantage of this method of skin protection.

Following completion of the surgical plan, the wound should be irrigated. Here, body temperature normal saline under moderate pressure (e.g., bulb syringe) is adequate. In contaminated areas, additional increase of irrigating fluid pressure can be achieved with commercially available systems. It is important, however, to remember that regardless of the pressure used with irrigation, only foreign bodies and surface contamination can be eliminated. It does not affect the interstitial bacterial count (as reflected by quantitative bacterial tissue analysis).

Any wound, expected to produce over 50 cc of drainage postoperatively, should be drained via a closed system. Also, any potential dead space or abscess site should be subjected to suction drainage. Judicial use of such a system is helpful to the wound-healing process by elimination of extravasated blood and other fluids. Any excessive amount of fibrin present in the wound (e.g., hematoma) slows down the wound-healing stages until the extravasated blood is eliminated through the process of natural degradation or surgical evacuation. The mechanical removal of hematoma is, of course, a matter of surgical judgment. The prolongation of wound healing is, however, only one aspect of the negative effect of hematoma. The expansion of the volume (even without any additional bleeding) is secondary to the hygroscopic nature of extravasated blood with its detrimental effect on the viability of the overlying tissue as well as an increase in concentration of free radicals. The availability of hematoma as a culture medium is self-evident.

Following wound closure, some form of a dressing is usually applied to the surgical site.

There are several reasons for doing that; collection of wound oozing, protection from patient and/or environment, compression, stabilization, and prevention of wound desiccation are the leading considerations. It is important, however, to realize that a wound closed primarily is considered watertight within the first 12 to 18 hours and thus protected from the environment. There are some potential drawbacks with dressings; interference with tissue vascularity when the dressing is too tight and delay in diagnosis of a hematoma or early infection are just a few. "Optimal" dressing should include a nonadherent layer (e.g., Xeroform), followed by a layer of an absorbent gauze, possibly even moist to increase its capillary absorbency, and, finally, a soft compressive layer (e.g., "fluffs") affixed with roll gauze. A tape should be laid on the dressing and not applied with stretch to prevent excessive compression (especially in children). Removal of this dressing can be done within several days, followed by the application of an antibacterial ointment. Any question regarding the wound status postoperatively should mandate immediate change of this dressing.

CHRONIC WOUNDS

Chronic wounds represent a significant interruption of the wound-healing process. This is usually due to the lack of adequate, well-oxygenated tissue available during an acute phase of wound healing or subsequent to a progressive deterioration of tissue blood supply.

The key to successful therapy of chronic wounds is the correct assessment of the biologic factors responsible for creating a chronic wound as well as timing of the therapeutic measures. In principle, some form of debridement of a wound is necessary with removal of the offending item, e.g., bony sequestrum, alloplastic material, or devitalized muscle, which then permit the interrupted healing phase to continue to completion.

Debridement assisted by enzymatic means, delivered as an external ointment, is usually minimally effective. Following surgical debridement, the use of wet-to-dry dressing (moist 4 × 4 gauze in normal saline applied directly to the wound and changed every 4 hours) is helpful when some drainage is present and additional "microscopic" debridement is performed (as

gauze dries up, small avascular tissue fragments adhere to it and are removed mechanically). In large wounds, additional coverage is usually required in the form of a flap.

Postradiation wounds pose a specific problem due to the extent of vascular damage to tissues at a great distance from the actual wound breakdown. Limited debridement, even when followed by bleeding from wound edges, is often followed by further necrosis. This could be explained on the basis of borderline capillary perfusion at the margins further embarrassed by surgical manipulation. The evidenced "bleeding" at the periphery often reflects vascular shunting that bypasses the capillary bed. It is better, in such situations, to plan on revascularizing the entire area with a flap right from the beginning.

A *granuloma* is usually considered to be a limited chronic wound. It is the end result of inflammation due to the presence of a foreign substance. Macrophages persist at the site of the injury when they are unable to make the material soluble. Fibroblasts also move into the area and surround the macrophages. Collagen is eventually deposited, enclosing the lesion in a dense, fibrous capsule forming a true granuloma. They can develop around nonabsorbable sutures and talcum from surgical gloves, among others.

Other types of foreign body reactions may be encountered, for example, with vascular grafts, silicone or methyl methacrylatic prostheses, and so on. The body interacts with any insoluble material either by extruding it, if it is mobile, by exposing (externalizing) it if it's close to the surface, or by walling it off by a process identical to granuloma formation. The intensity and the extent of the reaction, of course, varies widely, depending on the nature of the foreign body, patient's reactivity, and the soft tissue around it.

DENERVATED WOUNDS

The principal distinction of denervated skin from normal is the increased activity of collagenase in the denervated skin. In normal skin, collagenase is found in the dermis. In a healing wound, it is present also in the migrating epithelium and the underlying granulation tissue.

The normally present collagenase inhibitors in the serum prevent constant manifestation of this activity. Ischemia, even of short duration, eliminates the influence of collagenase inhibitors, permitting a full expression of abundance of collagenase in such a patient. This could explain massive decubiti occurring in paraplegic patients following minimal ischemia in contradistinction to those seen in debilitated patients with intact sensation.

Conclusion

Wound healing is as much a science as it is an art. Theoretical knowledge of the basic morphologic and biochemical events is essential to the rational understanding of various natural processes taking place following wounding. However, there is no substitution for the practical knowledge of wounds, which comes only from clinical experience, permitting us to "read" wounds at any given time. This assures the surgeon that he is in harmony with tissue biology and regional specificity in real time.

Acknowledgment

The author gratefully acknowledges the use of Earl Peacock's book *Wound Repair* in preparation of this chapter and encourages readers to refer to this textbook for a much more extensive summary of the wound-healing events.

Bibliography

David JC, Hunt TK (eds). Problem Wounds. The Role of Oxygen. New York: Elsevier Science Publishing, 1988.

Lineaweaver W, Howard R, Soucy D, et al. Topical antimicrobial toxicity. Arch Surg 1985;120:267–70 (reference for the detrimental affect of Betadine irrigation).

Peacock EE: Wound Repair. Philadelphia: W.B. Saunders, 1984.

Knighton DR, Silver IA, Hunt TK. Regulation wound healing angiogenesis—effective oxygen gradients and inspired oxygen concentration. Surgery 1981;90:262–70.

Ryan TJ (ed): New Insights into Wound Healing. Second International Forum, December 4, 1987. Amsterdam: Excerpta Medica, 1988.

T W O

ROBERT D. GOLDSTEIN, M.D.
BERISH STRAUCH, M.D.

Plastic Surgery Wound Coverage for the Neurosurgery Patient

The principles and techniques of plastic surgery are most often needed when there is soft tissue loss. In areas where the tissue loss is minimal, where there is skin laxity, or where there is no exposure of underlying vital structures (i.e., bones, joints, tendons, nerves, vessels, or viscera), wound closure is easily accomplished with simple or layered suturing of the wound. When this approach is not available, a variety of factors go into making the proper decision for wound closure. These include the status of the available blood supply at the site of tissue loss, the presence of contamination or infection, exposure of underlying vital structures, the need for pre and postoperative radiation, and the likelihood of having to perform secondary surgical procedures in the same operative field (Table 2–1).

Free Skin Grafts

Free skin grafting can be used to close any wound that has a blood supply sufficient to allow for inosculation (a spontaneous reconnection of the vasculature of the bed and the graft). Generally, this bed will develop spontaneous granulation tissue. Exceptions include bone denuded of periosteum, cartilage denuded of perichondrium, tendon denuded of peritenon, nerve denuded of perineurium, and heavily irradiated tissue. All of these areas are avascular and will not support a skin graft. Long-standing ulcers in chronic granulation tissue also serve as poorly vascularized beds.

Skin grafts when applicable can be used for permanent or temporary coverage. They are du-

15

Table 2-1.   Reconstructive Ladder
Illustrating Hierarchy of Wound Closure from
Simple to Complex

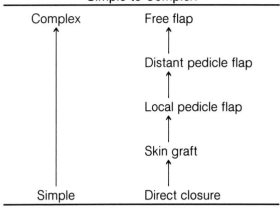

Complex	Free flap
	↑
	Distant pedicle flap
	↑
	Local pedicle flap
	↑
	Skin graft
	↑
Simple	Direct closure

rable when placed on a good padding of subcutaneous tissue or muscle. Skin grafts provide temporary coverage in a contaminated or irradiated area, or temporary coverage of some vital structure. They do not allow for the performance of secondary operative procedures beneath the graft, such as bone grafting or nerve grafting. Loss of the skin coverage would ensue.

A skin graft is a segment of dermis and epidermis that has been completely separated from its blood supply and donor site attachment before being transferred to another area of the body. Skin grafts can be classified as split-thickness grafts or full-thickness grafts. When they consist of epidermis and a portion of dermis, they are partial-thickness or split-thickness grafts. A full-thickness skin graft includes the entire dermis and epidermis (Fig. 2-1).

The split-thickness graft tends to be the most versatile and most popular. It is more likely to survive on its recipient site; the donor site will heal or reepithelialize more rapidly; and large amounts can be taken with little difficulty or morbidity. On the other hand, it will undergo a greater degree of soft tissue contracture. A thin graft will not transplant the hair follicles and sebaceous glands when transferred.

The split-thickness skin graft can be meshed. Meshing allows for increasing the area of coverage, allows the graft to conform to various contours of the body, and allows for egress of serum and blood during the healing process.

The full-thickness skin graft comprises the entire thickness of the skin. Because of its thickness, this skin graft is more slowly vascularized than the split-thickness graft, and therefore requires optimal conditions for a complete take. In addition, its characteristics approximate more closely those of normal skin than do those of the split-thickness graft. It has less of a tendency to undergo contracture and will generally give a superior cosmetic result (Table 2-2).

Although any area can serve as a donor site for a split-thickness graft, full-thickness grafts

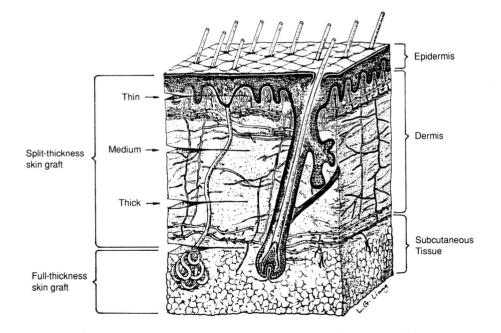

Figure 2-1.   Cross-section of skin illustrating relationship of epidermis and dermis to thickness of skin graft.

Table 2–2. Comparison of Split-Thickness Skin Graft and Full-Thickness Skin Graft

SPLIT-THICKNESS	FULL-THICKNESS
Better chance of take	More difficult take
More soft tissue contraction	Less soft tissue contraction
Less stable	More stable
Donor site healed by re-epithelialization	Donor site closed primarily
Large amounts available for harvest	Small amounts available
Retains fewer of the properties of donor skin	Retains more of the properties of donor skin

are most commonly taken from the retroauricular area, supraclavicular area, upper eyelid, intertriginous areas of the medial thigh, groin, or abdomen. All of these areas allow for primary closure of the donor site after harvesting the full-thickness graft.

In choosing the proper donor site for a full-thickness graft, one should consider skin color, texture, thickness, and hair-bearing nature of the donor site, because these areas will be transferred with the graft.

The care of any split-thickness skin graft must ensure that there is contact between the graft and the recipient bed. It is important to remove any clot or serum from the recipient bed before placing the graft and to evacuate any sera that may accumulate during the course of graft take. The skin graft may be cared for with either an open or a closed technique.

Skin grafts are not suitable in the following situations: (1) for covering of densely scarred areas or areas of functional stress; (2) for covering of bone with poor padding; (3) for covering tendons (tendons must be placed in a tissue that will allow gliding); (4) for covering of nerves (the skin graft may cause a scar contracture resulting in loss of conductivity, and the poor padding over the area of the nerve could lead to pain at the nerve site; and (5) for areas when secondary operations are necessary. An area in which an operation on bone, tendon, ligament, or joint is to be performed, or through which a peripheral nerve is to be explored, must be covered by a skin flap.

Flaps

When conditions dictate that a direct closure or skin graft are not appropriate, a flap will be needed. A flap is a unit of tissue that is transferred from a donor site to a recipient site while maintaining a continuous blood supply through a vascular pedicle. Flaps can be defined by either their blood supply or by their donor tissue. Those defined by their donor tissue (Fig. 2–2) can consist of cutaneous flaps, muscle flaps, myocutaneous flaps, osseocutaneous flaps, fasciocutaneous flaps, and omental flaps. Flaps defined by their blood supply come under the categories of random or local flaps, axial flaps, myocutaneous flaps, fasciocutaneous flaps, and free flaps.

The flap denotes the tissue and the pedicle denotes the point of attachment.

Skin Flaps

Skin flaps can be divided into two general types: random-pattern and those based on a definite arterial supply (Fig. 2–3). The random-pattern flap lacks a named anatomic arteriovenous system. These flaps receive their blood supply from segmental arteries that lie deep to the muscle, sending perforators at the flap base to a network in the dermal-subdermal plexus of the skin. Random-pattern flaps are limited by the length-to-width ratio of the tissue involved (1:1). Through the delay phenomenon, this 1:1 length-to-width ratio can be increased by as much as 60%. With this technique, the flap is developed and transferred in more than one stage. In the process, the blood supply through the subdermal plexus is reoriented and augmented, allowing the transfer of greater lengths of tissue. Random pattern flaps are more variable in their survival pattern.

Axial-pattern flaps contain at least one recognized arteriovenous system. These flaps receive their blood supply through a direct cutaneous artery that arises from an identifiable segmental axial artery by way of a perforating artery. The arterial flap consists of a proximal arterial pedicle and a more distal cutaneous random portion. When the skin is centered over a large cutaneous artery and vein, a flap of great length can be elevated, without the necessity of delayed tech-

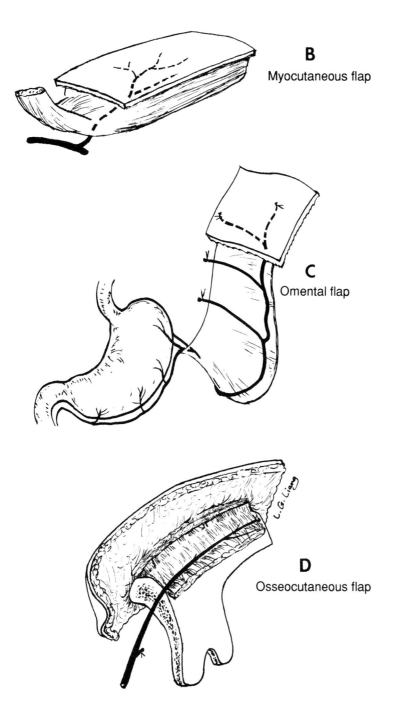

A
Cutaneous flap

B
Myocutaneous flap

C
Omental flap

D
Osseocutaneous flap

Figure 2-2.   Flaps defined by their donor tissue. **A:** cutaneous flap consisting of a vascular pedicle supplying skin and subcutaneous tissue; **B:** myocutaneous flap — the named vascular pedicle supplying a muscle and the overlying skin supplied by musculocutaneous perforator; **C:** omental flap; **D:** osseocutaneous flap — the named vascular pedicle supplies skin and bones.

Figure 2-3. Flaps defined by their blood supply. **A:** random pattern flap—circulation is supplied to the subdermal plexus via musculocutaneous perforator; **B:** axial pattern flap—a direct cutaneous axial vessel supplies a segment of skin and subcutaneous tissue without utilizing musculocutaneous perforator; **C:** myocutaneous flap—a named vessel provides circulation to a muscle and the overlying skin is supplied via the musculocutaneous perforator, providing for an entire skin muscle unit; **D:** fasciocutaneous flap—arterial trunk superficial to the deep fascia supplying the overlying skin. By including the deep fascia, a much longer flap can be created.

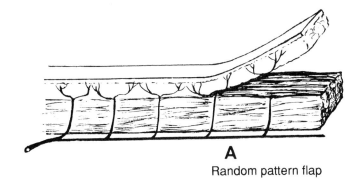

A

Random pattern flap

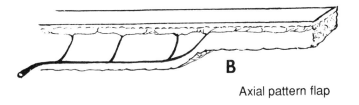

B

Axial pattern flap

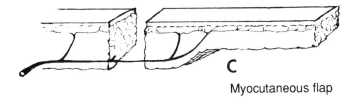

C

Myocutaneous flap

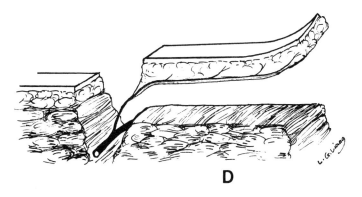

D

Fasciocutaneous flap

niques. Examples of these would include the deltopectoral flap, the groin flap, the superficial temporal artery flap, the dorsalis pedis flap, and the scapular flap.

A myocutaneous flap consists of a muscle and its attached overlying skin. Any muscle with a dominant vascular pedicle may be used as a myocutaneous flap. The various muscles of the body have a known arteriovenous system and the overlying skin, if attached to the muscle, receives its blood supply through interconnecting musculocutaneous perforators. When using a myocutaneous unit, care must be taken to preserve the integrity of the perforating musculocutaneous vessels between the muscle and the skin. Shearing forces during dissection can disrupt this vascular network.

The fasciocutaneous flap elevates skin with the underlying fascia and, as a result, a much longer flap can be developed. There are direct cutaneous vessels that run parallel to the skin immediately *above* the fascia. By elevating the skin and fascia, these vessels are included. This results in a flap with an augmented blood supply able to be safely developed, with length-to-width ratios of up to 3 : 1.

Osteocutaneous flaps are used when there is need to bridge large bone gaps. There are a number of areas that serve as sources of vascularized bone. Their requirements depend on the size of the bony defect, the shape of the bony defect, and the vascularity of the recipient bed. Sources of vascularized bone include the fibula with the peroneal artery, the iliac crest with the deep circumflex iliac artery, segments of the radius with the radial artery, segments of the scapula with the posterior circumflex scapular artery, and segments of the calverium with the superficial temporal artery. Each of these areas is also capable of transferring skin along with bone.

Classification for Random-Pattern Flaps

ROTATION FLAP

The rotation flap is a semicircular flap of skin and subcutaneous tissue that rotates about a pivot point into the defect to be closed (Fig. 2–4). Its donor site can be closed by a skin graft or by direct suturing of the wound. The line of

greatest tension in a rotation flap extends from the pivot point outward toward the most distant point of the defect.

TRANSPOSITION FLAP

The transposition flap is a rectangle or square of skin and subcutaneous tissue that also is rotated about a pivot point into an immediately adjacent defect (Fig. 2–5). By design, the end of the flap adjacent to the defect must extend beyond the defect. Then, as the flap is rotated into the line of greatest tension in the radius of the arc, the advancing tip of the flap will be sufficiently long. The flap donor site can be closed by skin grafting or direct suture of the wound.

INTERPOLATION FLAP

This flap consists of skin and subcutaneous tissue that is rotated in an arc about a pivot point into a nearby, but not immediately adjacent, defect (Fig. 2–6). The pedicle of this flap must therefore pass over or under intervening intact tissue. The flap donor site can be closed by skin grafts or direct suture of the wound.

ADVANCEMENT FLAP

This is a flap that moves into a defect without any rotation or lateral movement (Figs. 2–7, 2–8).

Tissue Expansion

The ability of tissue, especially skin, to stretch, is not novel. Advantages of tissue expansion are impressive: (1) tissue is made available from a local site; (2) color match and texture are better; (3) sensibility is preserved; and (4) there is no donor site that requires skin grafting. Disadvantages include: (1) multiple (at least two) surgical procedures; (2) multiple office visits for interval expansion; (3) pain during the expansion process; (4) risk of infection or extrusion of the expander; and (5) greater deformity during the final stages of the expansion.

The surgical technique involves the creation of a pocket for the Silastic expander adjacent to the defect. The deflated expander is placed in the pocket with an injection port situated in an

Figure 2–4. **A:** General schema of a rotation flap. **B:** Design of rotation flap for closure of scalp defect. Donor site would require skin graft. **C:** Double rotation flap S-plasty for closure of scalp defect.

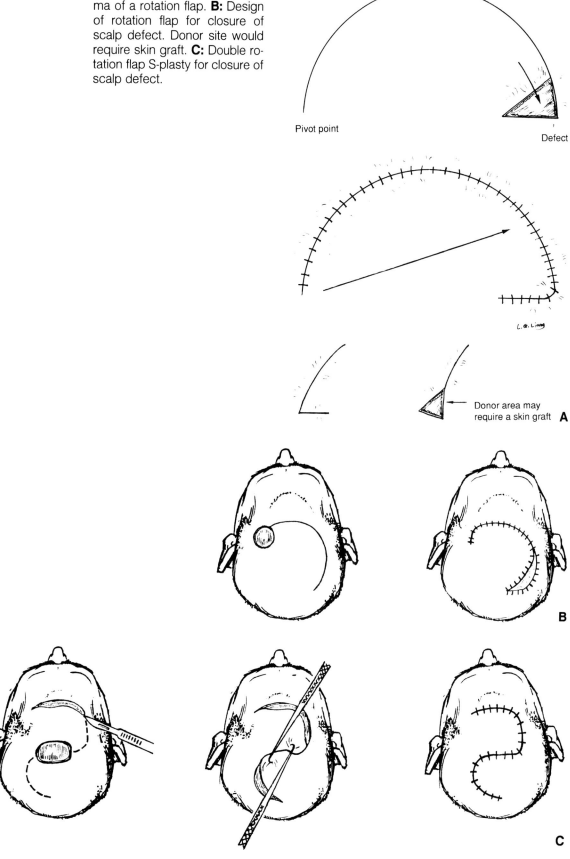

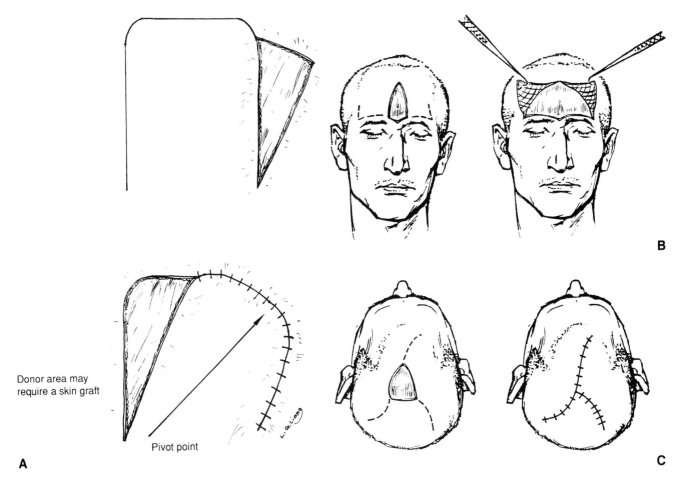

Figure 2–5.   **A:** Schema of transposition flap. **B:** Design of transposition flap with multiple incisions through undersurface of fascia to allow expansion of the flap. **C:** Gillies' tripod technique.

appropriate location. The surgical incision is allowed to heal, usually in 2 to 3 weeks. Over a period of weeks, under sterile conditions, increments of sterile saline are injected into the port, filling the expander and stretching the overlying skin. The rate of expansion is guided by the convenience of frequent visits, blood supply to the expanding skin, and local pain and discomfort.

Generally, neck and facial skin expand easily, with little discomfort. Scalp expansion tends to go slowly, and lower extremity skin expansion exhibits the greatest number of complications, especially related to infection and extrusion of the implant (Figs. 2–9, 2–10).

Surgical Anatomy of the Scalp

Superficial Temporal Fascia

The superficial temporal fascia (synonymous with temporal parietal fascia, epicranial aponeurosis, and galeal extension) is a thin, highly vascularized layer of connective tissue that lies immediately deep to the hair follicles (Fig. 2–11). It is continuous with the galea above, the frontalis muscle in front, the occipitalis muscle behind, and the superficial musculo-aponeurotic system (SMAS) layer of the face below. The plane of

Figure 2-6. Interpolation flap.

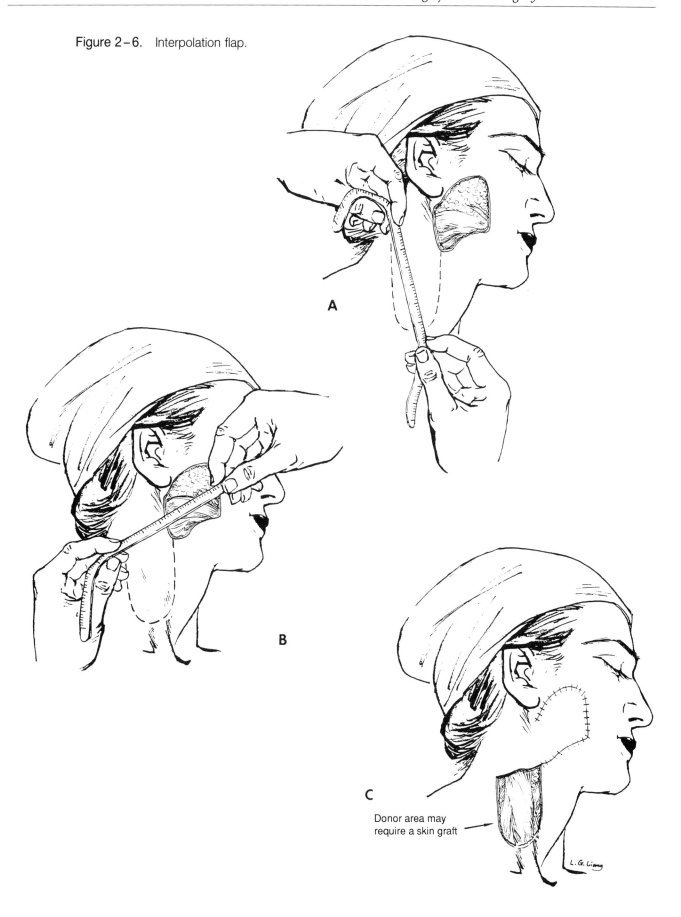

Donor area may
require a skin graft

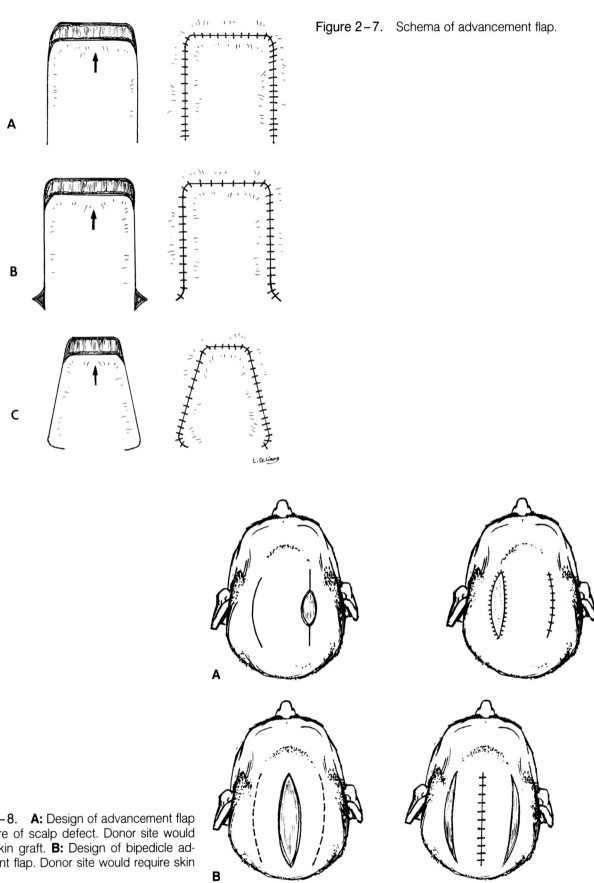

Figure 2–7.   Schema of advancement flap.

Figure 2–8.   **A:** Design of advancement flap for closure of scalp defect. Donor site would require skin graft. **B:** Design of bipedicle advancement flap. Donor site would require skin graft.

Figure 2–9. **A,B,C:** A 4-year-old girl with large bony deformity of spine. Two months prior to kyphectomy, four tissue expanders were inserted to stretch the surrounding skin and allow for skin closure at the time of bony resection.

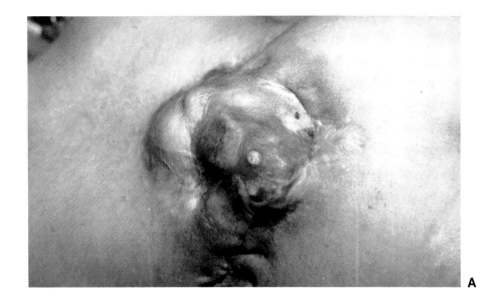

A

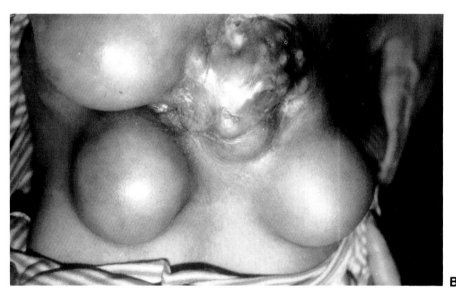

B

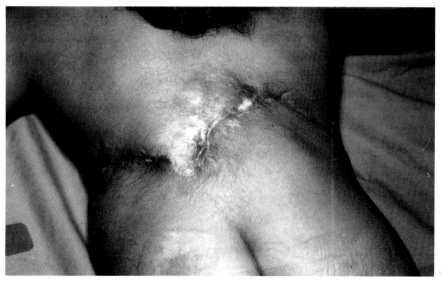

C

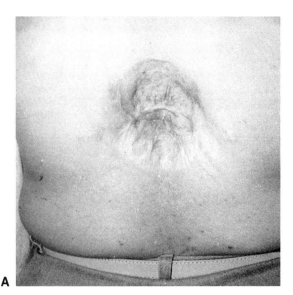

Figure 2–10. **A,B,C:** A 40-year-old woman with painful skin graft on her back placed after removal of skin tumor. Tissue expansion allowed for removal of the skin graft.

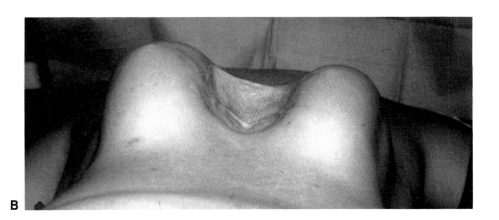

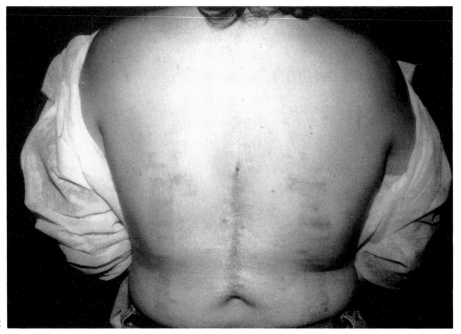

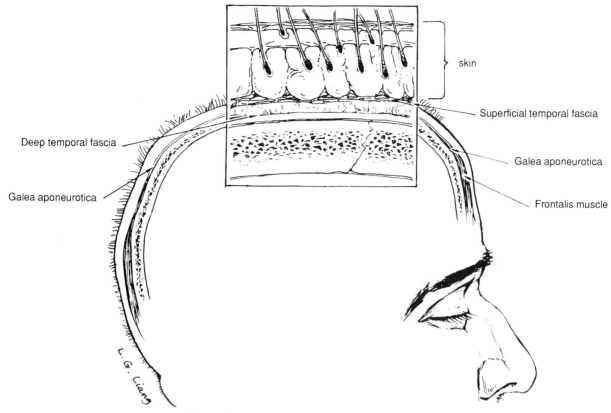

Figure 2–11.   Surgical anatomy of the scalp.

dissection is immediately deep to the hair follicles. Its blood supply is the superficial temporal artery and vein. The artery and vein lie at slightly different levels: the vein lies right below the hair follicles on the outer surface of the fascia; the artery lies within the thickness of the fascia.

The superficial temporal artery divides into an anterior and posterior division, about 2 cm above the zygomatic arch. After this, the branching is irregular.

Galea Aponeurotica

This connects the top of the occipitalis muscle with the top of the frontalis muscle. The galea and the superficial temporal fascia are names for neighboring parts of the same layer.

Subaponeurotic Plane

The superficial temporal fascia is separated from the deep temporal fascia by a distinct layer of loose areolar tissue. No vessels cross this plane. It is this plane that gives the scalp its natural mobility.

Deep Temporal Fascia

This is a dense, tough layer that invests the temporalis muscle and ends with an attachment of the deep temporal fascia to the periosteum. The deep temporal fascia receives its blood supply from the middle temporal artery, a branch of the superficial temporal artery.

Coverage of Scalp Defects

Scalp defects with intact periosteum will readily accept a skin graft (Fig. 2–12). If the outer table of the skull is devoid of periosteum, a skin graft will not take, and a flap is required (Figs. 2–13, 2–14). The superficial temporal fascia (galea) is a dense layer that limits the elasticity of the scalp. Multiple superficial incisions through the undersurface of the superficial temporal fascia (galea) permit advancement and extension of

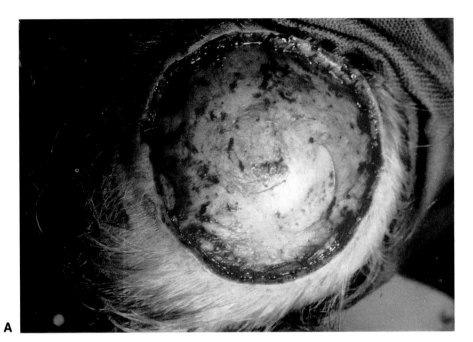

A

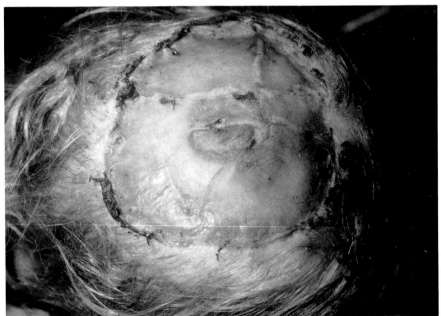

B

Figure 2–12. **A,B:** Scalp defect with intact periosteum and healed skin graft.

the tissue (Fig. 2–15). Orticochea has devised a three- and four-flap method for closure of moderate-size defects (Figs. 2–16, 2–17). With this technique it may be necessary to score the undersurface of the flaps to allow for expansion.

Back Defects

Tissue available for closure of back defects includes a variety of local flaps, musculocutaneous flaps, and soft tissue expansion. Defects of the upper third of the back are within the territory of the trapezius and latissimus dorsi muscles; the middle third is within the territory of the latissimus dorsi muscle; and the lower third is within the territory of the gluteus maximus muscle (Fig. 2–18).

The latissimus dorsi muscle can be used as a sliding advancement flap (Fig. 2–19) as for a myelomeningocele (Fig. 2–20) or as a transposition flap as for closure of a radiation ulcer to the back. (The reader will also find further discussion of myelomeningocele repair in Chapter 4.)

Figure 2-13. **A,B,C:** Scalp defect devoid of periosteum requiring a local flap.

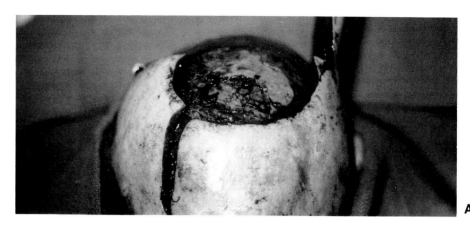

A

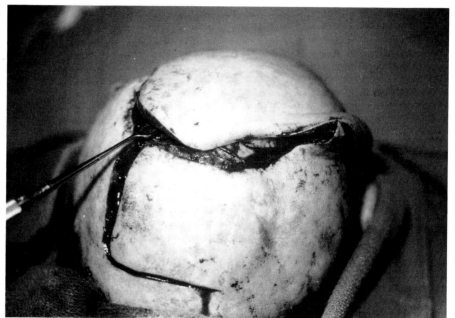

B

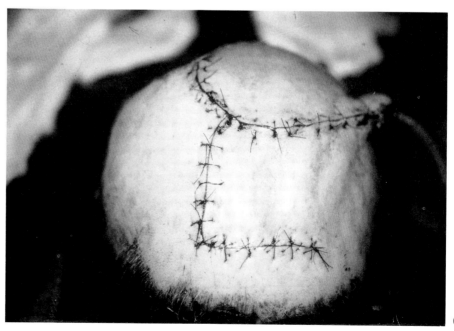

C

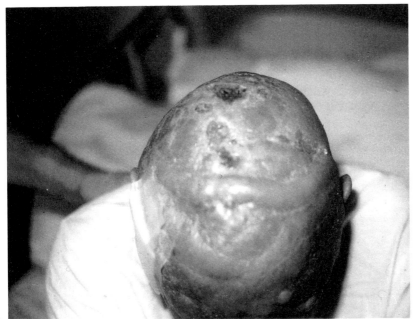

A

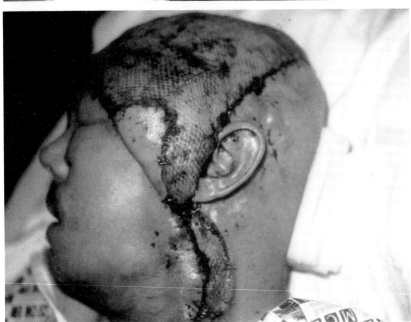

B

Figure 2–14. **A,B:** Extensive lymphoma of scalp requiring complete excision and coverage with latissimus dorsi free flap.

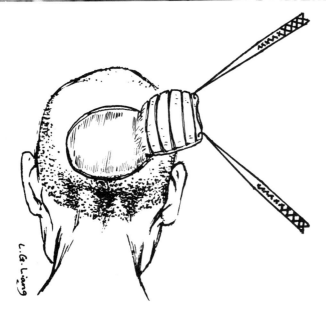

Figure 2–15. Multiple incision through the undersurface of the superficial temporal fascia permits expansion of the flap.

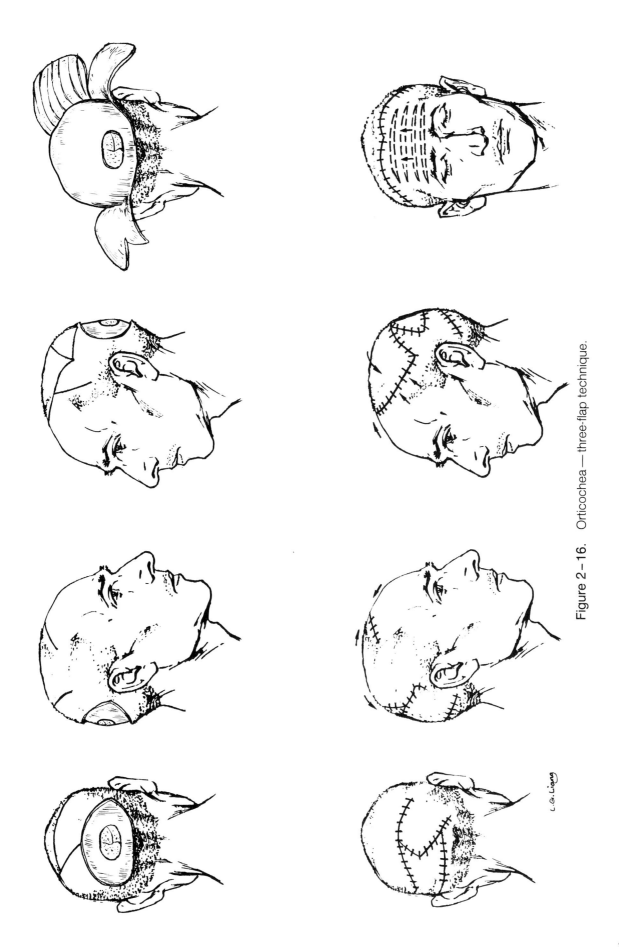

Figure 2–16. Orticochea — three-flap technique.

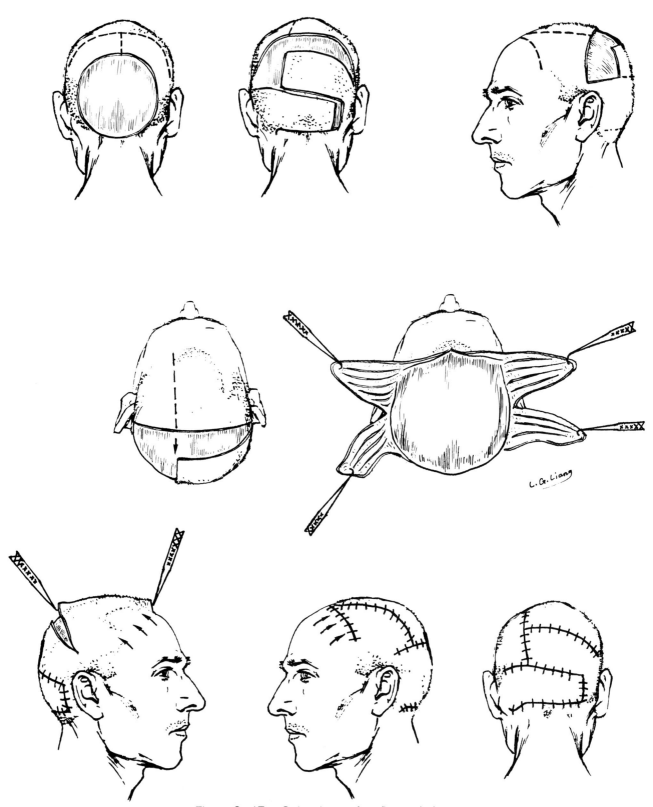

Figure 2–17.   Orticochea — four-flap technique.

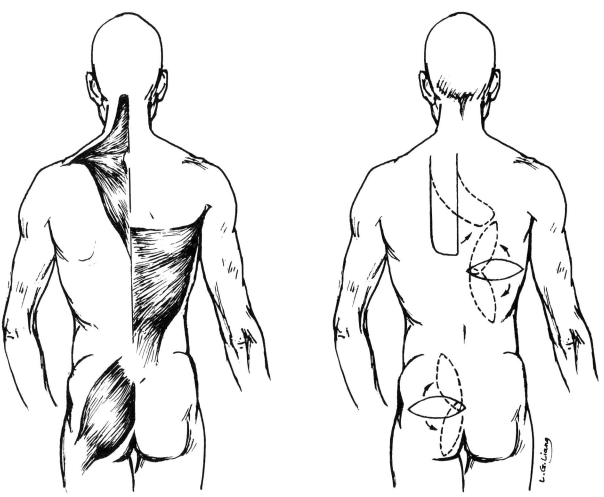

Figure 2–18.   Myocutaneous flaps available for soft tissue defects of the back.

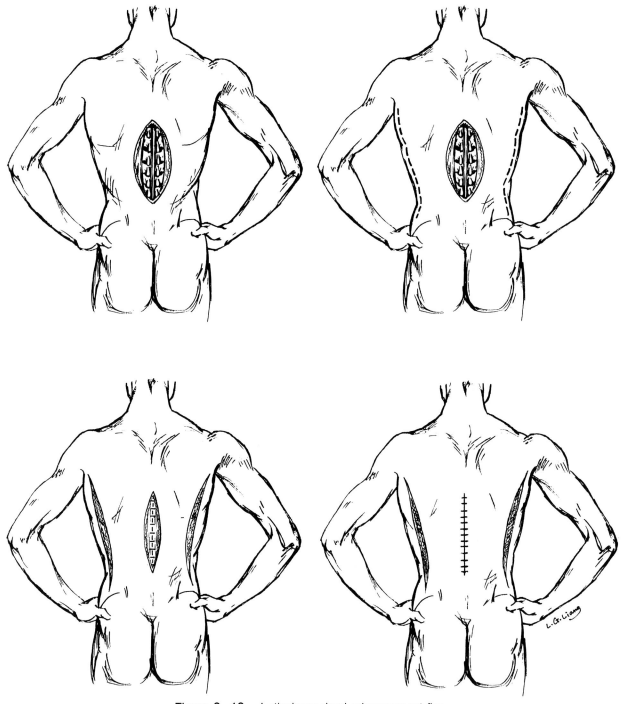

Figure 2–19.   Latissimus dorsi advancement flap.

The trapezius flap can be oriented vertically or horizontally and the gluteal flap can be used as a rotation advancement flap.

The principles involved in choosing a safe and appropriate wound closure are directed by local factors (radiation, contamination, exposure of vital structures) and the possible need for future surgery in the area (bone grafting or bone resection, nerve grafts, etc.) With the knowledge of the regional vascular anatomy and principles of moving tissue as skin grafts or flaps, the surgeon can make the correct decision for closure of simple and complex wounds.

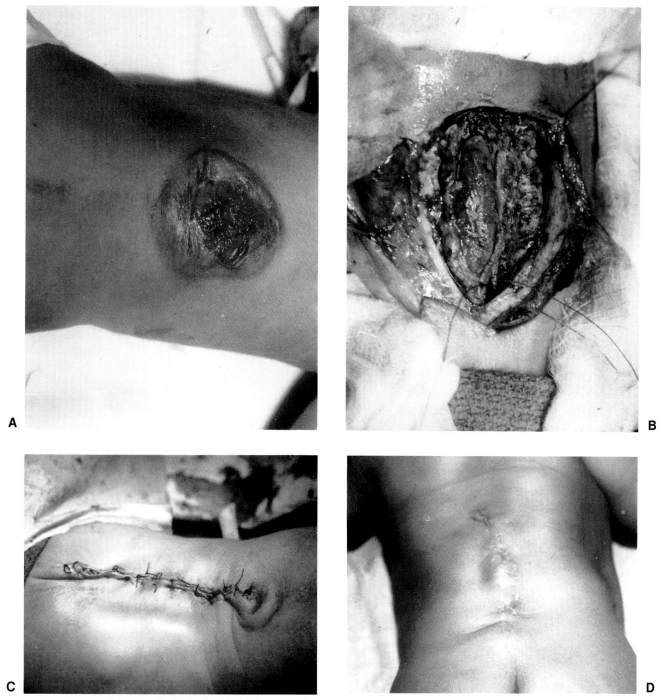

Figure 2–20.   **A–D:** Use of latissimus dorsi myocutaneous advancement flap for closure of myelo-meningocele.

Bibliography

Abul-Nassan HS, Van Drase Ascher G, et al. Surgical anatomy and blood supply of the fascial layer of the temporal region. Plast Reconstr Surg 1986;117:17–28.

Argenta LC, Austad ED. Tissue expansion. Clin Plast Surg 1987;14:3.

Barclay TL, Cardoso E, Sharpe DT, Crockett DJ. Repair of lower leg injuries with fasciocutaneous flaps. Br J Plast Surg 1982;35:126–32.

Brent B. Experience with the temporoparietal fascial free flap. Plast Reconstr Surg 1985;76:177–188.

Converse JR (ed). Reconstructive Plastic Surgery, 2nd ed. Philadelphia: W.B. Saunders, 1977: vol I, pp 152–239; vol II, pp 822–57.

Grabb WC, Smith JW (eds): Plastic Surgery. Boston: Little, Brown, 1979, pp 3–74, 265–79.

Mathes SJ, Nahai F (eds). Clinical Applications for Muscle and Musculocutaneous Flaps. St. Louis: C.V. Mosby, 1982.

Mathes SJ, (moderator): Symposium on Musculocutaneous Flaps. Contemp Surg 1985;26:85–117.

Porter B: The fasciocutaneous flap: Its use in soft tissue defects of the lower leg. Br J Plast Surg 1981;34:215–20.

Vasconez L, Mathes SJ, Gant TD: Musculocutaneous flaps in reconstructive surgery. Contemp Surg 1976;14:15–26.

THREE

CRAIG D. HALL, M.D.
JAMES T. GOODRICH, M.D., PH.D.

Repair of Calvarial Bone Defects: Cranioplasty and Bone–Harvesting Techniques

Cranioplasty simply defined is the reconstruction of a cranial defect. When the neurosurgeon replaces a bone flap at the end of a craniotomy, a cranioplasty has been performed. However, in our minds, we create a temporal separation of a craniotomy closure from a cranioplasty: cranioplasty thus becomes restricted to reconstructions of cranial defects.

The temporal element assumes the greatest significance because the original autogenous bone flap no longer exists; therefore a replacement must be fabricated. The scalp, often from previous surgery, infection, or trauma, is scarred, attenuated, and otherwise adherent to underlying dura. Thus, a cranioplasty, because of its temporal delay, becomes a sequenced reconstruction: first, the separation of dura from its overlying scar plane; second, the fabrication of a cranial substitute; and third, the provision of a well-vascularized soft tissue cover. The successful cranioplasty demands that each of these three preconditions be satisfied.

Indications and Timing

Cranial defects have assuredly existed since primitive man first trephined in search of cure, and probably prior to this event. Additionally, the use of coconut shells by South Sea islanders guarantees that man has probably been performing cranioplasties for an equivalent length of time.[1] These early efforts to repair cranial defects represent both functional and aesthetic desires.

Functionally, an intact skull represents a protective barrier against inadvertent blunt or penetrant trauma. The lower limit of defect size expressing functional concern is established by palpation. Therefore defects of greater than 2 cm and not underlying temporalis or occipitalis muscles are indications from a functional standpoint. An additional caveat is: any cranial defect in a patient who suffers from a seizure disorder should be considered a functional indication.

Aesthetically, the indications are set by visual criteria, so any defect of the frontoglabellar region or cranial convexity with a perceived loss of contour expands on the functional criteria. Given these broad guidelines, exclusion from cranioplastic reconstruction includes hydrocephalus, autoinfection, and contaminated wounds.

Cranial defects occur from traumatic, congenital, acquired, and infectious etiologies. The etiologic cause of the cranial defect directly affects the timing of the cranioplasty. Compound, penetrating traumatic and infection defects are best delayed 1 year—a guideline established by Rish et al.[2] in a cooperative study of 491 cranioplasties—acute repairs risking infection from immediate contamination and repairs prior to 1 year risking infection from organisms sequestered within the scar bed. Defects related to congenital or acquired etiologies need not be delayed. Timing in these cases is governed solely by the medical status of the patient.

Preparation of the Cranial Defect

The preparation of the cranial defect is technically constant, regardless of the cranioplastic technique selected. Preparation is predicated on solid surgical tenets: (1) maintenance of well-vascularized bed and flap; (2) gentle handling of tissues; (3) removal of all foreign bodies; and (4) hemostasis. Among these tenets, the most crucial to successful cranioplasties is the deliberate provision and maintenance of well-vascularized tissue.

The vast majority of cranioplasties are performed following previous trauma and/or surgery (Figs. 3–1, 3–2). These previous tissue in-

sults have led to scarring, attenuation of tissue, and limited vascular territories. As discussed in Chapter 2, preoperative planning must assess the scalp for the position of previous scars, the remaining regional blood supply, and the available tissue for transposition or rotation. In repetition of general principles, the surgeon should avoid the creation of parallel scars, incisions overlying the defect to be reconstructed, division of major vascular branches, and transgressions into nonhair-bearing areas.

Gentle handling of tissues requires that the scalp flap overlying the cranial defect be elevated with care, lest inadvertent dural penetration occurs. Similarly, surrounding paracranial flaps may be elevated with saline irrigation and broad, rounded periosteal elevators. Paracranial flaps supply additional vascularized coverage and are of critical importance when cranial defects are contiguous with sinus spaces.

Removal of foreign bodies in cranioplasty refers to the obliteration of mucosa from sinus spaces, debridement of devascularized tissue, and the creation of fresh, bleeding bone edges at the site of the cranial defect. Sinus spaces, once stripped of their mucosa, must be covered by vascularized, viable paracranial flaps prior to starting reconstruction of the defect. Loose bone chips, devascularized soft tissue, and desiccated paracranium increase the risk of infection by providing a safe harbor for bacteria.

A sharp curette may be used along the margins of the cranial defect to clear parasitic soft tissue from the underlying dura. Freshening the bony edges of the cranial defect is accomplished with a high-speed burr. Only the external table of bone need be cleared to assure a viable bony margin.

Having prepared the cranial defect in this manner, any of the following cranioplastic reconstructions may be undertaken.

Autogenous Bone Cranioplastic Reconstructions

The experience of plastic surgery in developing usable autogenous tissue for reconstruction of the body is readily transferable to a neurosurgical discipline. The three areas of autogenous bone under discussion are the bilamellar tem-

Figure 3–1. Typical example of a traumatic injury to the left frontal region with a resultant large defect in the calvarium and temporal region.

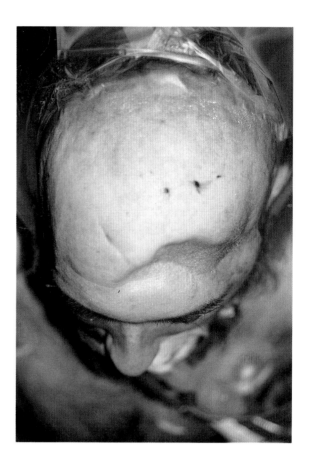

Figure 3–2. Three-dimensional CT reconstruction showing the frontal defect — a most helpful diagnostic aid in planning the surgical reconstructions.

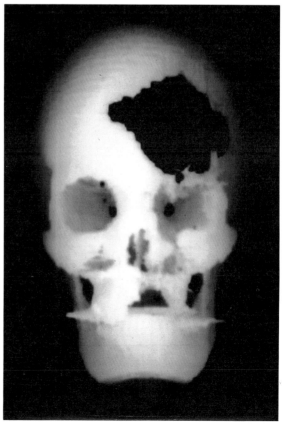

plate of the skull itself, costochondral rib grafts, as well as iliac crest and table grafts. The advantages of autogenous bone grafting are that the patient's own biomaterials are used for the reconstruction: this means that the availability of the autogenous bone is limited by the patient's donor resources and by the surgeon's expertise in obtainment.

Autogenous bone is superior to synthetic substitutes, in that it is readily incorporated into the patient's existing bony matrix, being a natural biologic material. Its adherence to soft tissue is inherently greater than that of any artificial substitute, lessening the potential risk of infections, and allowing remodeling of the autogenous bone by the overlying soft tissue forces.

Autogenous Cranial Bone Cranioplasty

The use of autogenous cranial bone for cranioplasty presents the surgeon with a dual challenge of design and procurement. Issues of design relate to cranial bone rigidity, thereby necessitating that a near mirror image of the cranial defect be located along the contour of the patient's cranium. Locating the cranial donor site is best accomplished by preparing a template of the cranial defect (Fig. 3–3). Our choice of template material is aluminum foil or aluminum wire, since both are malleable and will hold

a curvilinear form; however, latex and paper templates have both been used without significant difficulty. Care should be taken to assure that the outlined template is approximately 4 to 5 mm larger than the cranial defect. Given the bilamellar nature of the cranial bone, the internal table, because of its smaller arc size, requires the increased diameter of bone harvest, since the template has been marked on the external table.

Once formed, the template is "walked" over the surface of the cranium until a region of complimentary curvature and surface area is encountered (see Fig. 3–3). Small cranial defects may obviously be satisfied by using the inherent symmetry of the contralateral pericranium. Defects that cross the midline present greater topologic challenges.

Having satisfied the challenge of design, the procurement of the donor bone flap remains. The donor bone flap is elevated using standard craniotomy techniques, taking care to assure that in cases of continuity between defect and donor site, stable margins are preserved for cranial fixation (Fig. 3–4). Once harvested, the bilamellar cranial plate is split, using an air-driven reciprocating saw (Figs. 3–5, 3–6). Care must be taken to water cool the flap during the saw cuts to prevent thermal injury to the bone flap. Final separation of the internal from external lamella often requires the use of curved osteotomes to complete the intradiploic osteotomy.

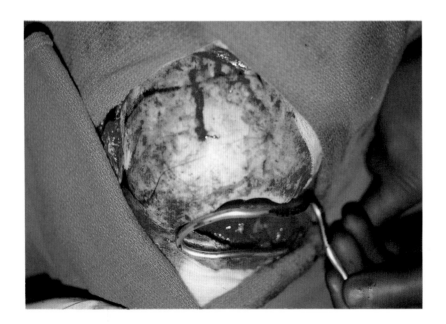

Figure 3–3. After a bifrontal skin flap is turned, the trauma site is fully exposed. Using a template, in this case a soft malleable aluminum wire, the site to be repaired is marked out. By "walking" the template over the exposed normal calvarium, a piece of corresponding size calvarium is located. We have marked out the craniotomy donor site in blue in this photograph.

Figure 3–4. The craniotomy has been completed and the calvarial bone to be split is shown here lifted out of the donor site.

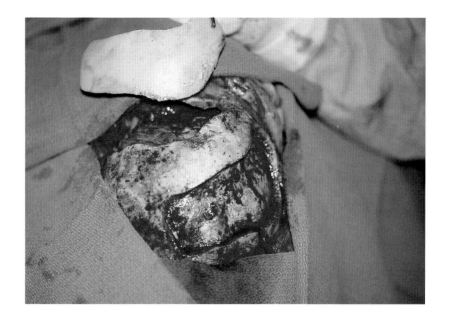

Figure 3–5. The surgeon is splitting the donor bone along the inner table using a reciprocating saw. Constant irrigation must be applied, and because of the translucent nature of the bone, it is easy to follow the diploic plane. It is important to try and keep both bone units of the same thickness. The inner table will then be placed back in the donor site. The outer table is used as the graft unit.

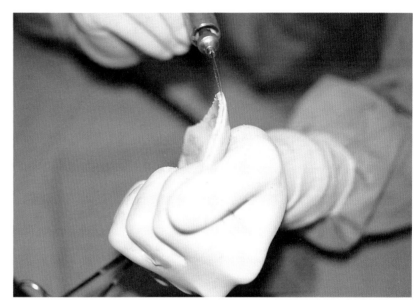

Figure 3–6. This figure shows the two units of calvarial bone after the diploic split.

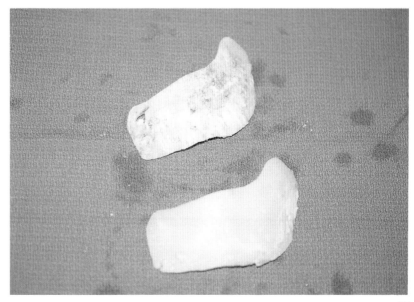

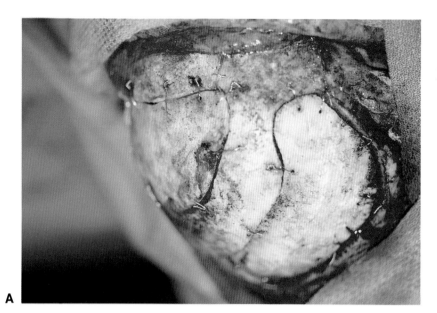

A

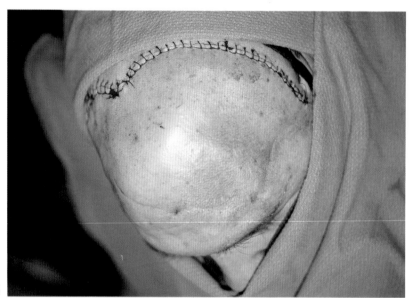

B

Figure 3–7. **A, B:** Operative photographs after placement of the two units. It is easy to appreciate here the symmetry and aesthetic reconstruction that is obtainable using this technique.

Once separated, the external bony lamella is returned to the original donor site, being stabilized with interosseous wire fixation. The internal lamella acts as the true autogenous cranial bone graft. Despite the template, controlled localization of donor site secondary contouring of the cranial graft is occasionally necessary. Surface irregularities can be remodeled using a high-speed water-cooled burr. Curvature discrepancies are best handled by making radial cuts in the margin of the bone plate, thereby allowing flattening and expansion to occur (Fig. 3–7).

Small cranial defects of 3 × 3 cm or less have been reconstructed by the authors without a formal craniotomy. In these cases, because of the small surface area involved, the convexity of the defect assumes less importance. Once again, a template of the defect is made and transferred to a neighboring parietal region. Once marked, a high-speed burr is used to create a trough surrounding the pattern. The trough is taken down to bleeding diploe. Smoothing of the outer edges of the trough is performed with a flat burr (Fig. 3–8). A flat reciprocating saw blade can then be used to split the lamellas of the

Figure 3-8. Donor site exposed on the calvarium. Here the bone grooves have been made with the beveled outer table evident.

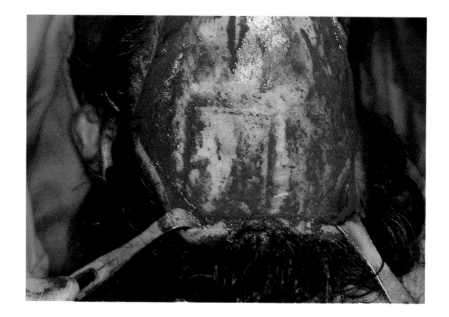

Figure 3-9. The saw is in position and one can easily remove the outer table of bone. A simple technique when a craniotomy is not required, but one can still harvest a reasonably good sized piece of donor bone.

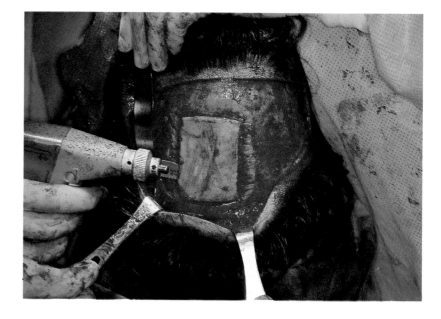

cranial bone, removing the external table and leaving the internal table intact (Fig. 3-9). This procedure is best performed on the parietal plate immediately superior to the origin of the temporalis muscle. After successfully removing the outer table, the edges of the donor harvest site are again contoured with an air-cooled burr to flatten the transition zone, thereby eliminating a palpable shelf (Fig. 3-10). The external table is then transferred to the previously prepared cranioplasty site and affixed with stainless steel wires.

Success of the procedure is dependent on adequacy of soft tissue coverage, and healthy, viable galeal flaps should be brought into apposition overlying both the donor and recipient sites. Closed suction draining is recommended, but this is left to the preference of the operating surgeon.

Complications with this outlined procedure have been less then 5%, and most of the complications have been related to small postoperative hematomas and seroma collections. The incidence of infection in our hands has been 1%.

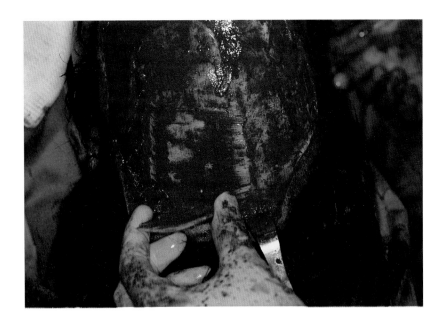

Figure 3–10. The outer table being elevated.

Again, the split cranial bone graft represents the state of the art in cranioplasties, providing the patient with one autogenous tissue of native membranous bone for the reconstruction that will be rapidly incorporated, rigid, will go on to bony union, and will be successful in remodeling, according to the soft tissue stresses placed above it.

Costochondral Rib Grafts

Costochondral rib grafts are readily available to the surgeon. In any surgical position required by the neurosurgical operation, they can be harvested in a posterior, lateral, or anterior format: anteriorly, because of the position of the breast and chest wall, it is conventional to choose the fourth and sixth ribs; posteriorly, because of limitations of the positions of the scapula, the eighth, ninth, and tenth ribs are convenient. In a lateral position with the arm abducted anteriorly, the fourth through eighth ribs can easily be excised.

Once again, the cranial defect for reconstruction has been freed of its dural attachments, creating a free edge of the cranial defect. The

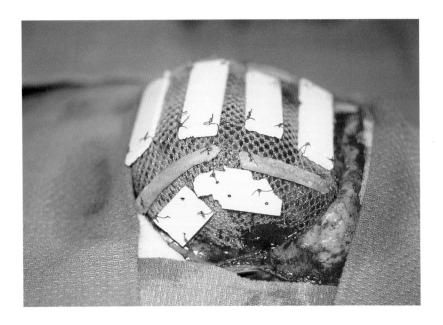

Figure 3–11. An operative example where only the lattice network is used; here the split rib grafts are supplemented with hydroxyapatite. We have used an underlying Dacron mesh to act as a strut support for various materials.

split costal bone graft is then measured to size, overcorrecting by 5 mm, and its curvature corrected. The resultant ends of the costochondral graft are wired into position on the cranial bone.

Munro and Guyuron[3] reported in the June 1981 issue of *Annals of Plastic Surgery* a method of latticework reconstruction that they described as the "wire-link fence," in which the split costal bone is woven, much as one would weave a basket, interlacing multiple segments of rib graft and wiring this woven latticework to the free edges of the cranial bone (Fig. 3–11).

Despite its ready availability, costochondral rib graft is a secondary bone choice compared with cranial bone, because costochondral rib graft has been shown through numerous studies to undergo substantial resorption, compared with that of membranous bone of the cranium.[4] The difference between the rates of resorption is believed to be secondary to an inherent difference between the receptivity of membranous bone for revascularizing versus that of endochondral bone.

The harvesting of costochondral graft will be described for an anterior position, but the techniques are readily transferable to lateral or posterior approaches. The procedure is initiated by establishing the rib to be harvested, by counting from the sternal angle of Louis representing the second rib space landmark. The ribs are then counted sequentially, starting from the second rib down. In males, any rib inferior to the free

edge of the pectoralis muscle can be used as a potential rib for harvesting. In females, the inframammary crease is the fixed anatomic landmark for deciding which is the most appropriate rib for harvest. Anteriorly, these usually represent the fourth and sixth ribs.

The procedure commences by incising through skin and subcutaneous tissue. Traditionally, a 4-cm transverse incision is required directly over the midportion of the rib. On reaching the muscular fascia, electrocoagulation is used to divide the fascial and muscular fibers down to the periosteum of the rib. The periosteum of the rib is incised with a scalpel blade. A Key periosteal elevator is used to raise the anterior periosteum from the rib. An Alexander periosteal elevator is then used to strip the superior and inferior free borders of the rib, starting medially and extending laterally. Once these have been stripped, a pigtail periosteal elevator is used to complete the separation of the periosteum, taking care that on the deep surface of the rib, periosteum overlying the parietal pleura is kept intact.

By separating off the entire periosteal envelope from the rib, the integrity of the thoracic space is maintained and the risk of pneumothorax minimized. Additionally, the preservation of the periosteal envelope allows for regeneration of a rudimentary rib. This rib regeneration occurs approximately 6 months postoperatively.

A full anterior resection of the costal bone

Figure 3–12. Splitting a rib using an osteotome.

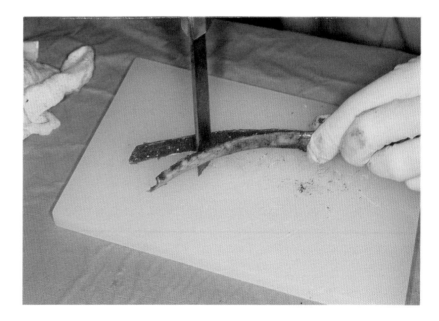

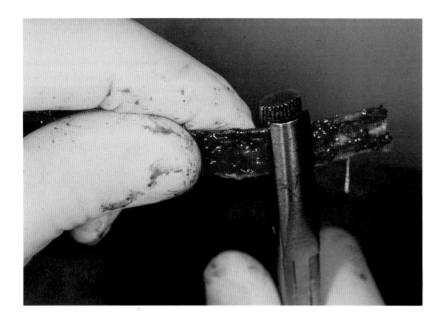

Figure 3–13. Bending into shape a split rib using a Tessier rib bender.

graft extends from the junction of the costo-chondral "synchondrosis" anteriorly to the posterior axillary line that represents the "transverse process," the angular portion of the rib. A right-angle bone cutter is then inserted into the periosteal pocket, and the synchondrosis of the costochondral junction is divided first, allowing elevation of the rib and creating an increased space in the periosteal pocket for the posterior osteotomy. Sections of rib up to 7 cm in length can be delivered through this approach.

Once harvested, the costal graft is split, using a sharp, straight 4-mm osteotome along the free superior or inferior borders (Fig. 3–12). This maneuver is best done by hand without the use of a mallet, since use of a mallet frequently leads to slippage of the osteotome and premature fracture of the rib. Once split, the rib can be recontoured using a Tessier rib bender (Fig. 3–13). This allows the convexity of the rib to be flattened or increased, depending on the operative needs of the surgeon.

The donor site is closed in layers: first, by reapproximating the periosteal layer, followed by the musculofascial layer, and then a two-layered closure of the chest wall. The use of a closed system drain is infrequent in harvesting costochondral grafts, particularly when electro-diathermy is used for control of hemostasis. The more frequent complication of pneumothorax can be treated by placement of a 10 F red rubber tube into the pleural defect, and closure of the pleural defect with an absorbable suture during a Valsalva maneuver. The red rubber tube is then put to low water-sealed suction; approximately 20 cc of water pressure is applied. When the patient is in the recovery room, once a chest x-ray has established the absence of a pneumothorax, the red rubber tube is removed and an occlusive dressing of petrolatum gauze and plain gauze is placed over the wound.

The incidence of pneumothoraces in our experience of elevating costochondral grafts carries a relative risk of 3%, given that no effort is made to separate the cartilaginous portion of the costochondral structure.

Incisions placed in the inframammary crease of the female patient heal well, without visible scarring. In the male patient, because of the tendency for traction by the pectoralis muscle, there is a small tendency toward spread scarring.

In summary, the benefits of rib autogenous bone graft are its availability of procurement in prone, supine, or lateral positions, and its ability to be easily curved and contoured. The limitations of rib graft cranioplasties are their tendency to undergo a sizeable degree of resorption that may lead to late contour irregularities, and their distant donor site.[5]

Iliac Bone Grafting

The iliac crest and dual tables of the ilium itself represent a tertiary source of bone for an autogenous reconstruction. Once again, the hierarchy regarding autogenous bone would be: cranial bone first, followed by costal bone, and the ilium as a third option. The iliac bone is similar to costochondral rib graft, being of endochondral origin and therefore having a greater rate of resorption than cranial bone, as mentioned previously for costal bone.

The uniqueness of the ilium rests on its ability to provide a flat, curved table of unilamellar or bilamellar bone, along with an additional source of cancellous bone. Being of autogenous nature, it has similar benefits to costal bone. The distinct advantage is that it does not offer the complication of pneumothoraces; however, there is muscle spasm of the pelvic girdle and limitation of ambulation for approximately 3 to 4 weeks postoperatively.

The approach to harvesting iliac table bone is as described by Tessier.[6] The superficial landmarks are those of the iliac crest. The anterosuperior iliac spine is located and marked with an X. A line is drawn with skin-marking pen along the superior iliac crest. To avoid painful scar and hypertrophic scar formation, the line of incision is placed 1 to 2 cm below the level of the iliac crest. Once this has been marked out with a skin pen, the transverse width of the incision is usually on the order of 4 cm.

Surgery is begun by elevating the lateral thigh skin to the level of the iliac crest. The initial incision is made through skin and subcutaneous tissue, down to the muscular fascial aponeurosis of the external oblique as it inserts on the iliac crest. The aponeuroses of the internal and external oblique muscles are then incised down to the transversalis fascia. This incision allows the transversalis to be separated from the internal table of the iliac in a subperiosteal plane, mobilizing the abdominal wall contents medially away from the internal table of the iliac.

Deaver retractors or broad-base Tessier retractors are then used to provide exposure of the field. If cancellous bone is the requirement for the case, the iliac crest can be distracted in the following manner. An oscillating saw is used to create two transverse cuts along the iliac crest, carrying them down approximately 2 cm into the substance of the iliac wing. A right-angle oscillating saw is then used to create an osteotomy along the internal table of the iliac bone, connecting the two transverse osteotomies. An osteotome is then used to complete these osteotomies and Kocher clamps used to out-fracture the iliac crest laterally, keeping its periosteal blood supply from the gluteus maximus and lateral thigh abductors intact (Fig. 3–14).

With the cancellous space exposed, the cancellous bone can then be harvested using variable-sized curettes. The entire cancellous volume of the ilium can be removed through this approach without difficulty, and generates up to 20 cc of bone volume in an adult patient.

The more frequent source for cortical table reconstruction uses the same approach with transposition of the iliac crest. The 90° oscillating saw for cortical bone harvest outlines the

Figure 3–14. An incision has been made over the iliac crest and after harvesting the cancellous bone it is being lifted out.

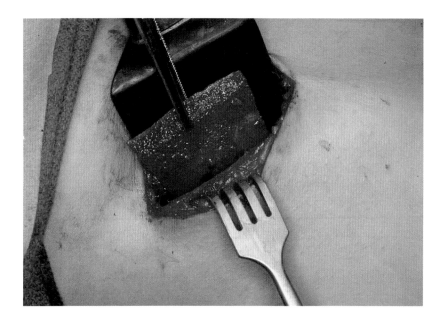

rectangular plate of inner table. The saw osteotomy is in the shape of the cranioplast template. After performing the osteotomy of the internal table, a 4 to 6 mm osteotome is placed within the cancellous bone space; a mallet is used, as necessary, to complete the osteotomy. Then, gentle out-fracture of the segment allows delivery of an intact inner table of iliac bone.

Surgicel treated with thrombin can be used to pack the cancellous space of the iliac bone to provide hemostasis postoperatively. It is frequently necessary to use a closed-suction drain to prevent hematoma formation and muscle spasm in the postoperative period. The wound is closed in layers in the following manner.

A through-and-through 1-0 Vicryl suture is used to pass through the periosteal hinge of the iliac crest. The same suture then passes through the external fascia of the gluteus maximus and is finished by attaching to the aponeurosis of the external and internal oblique, thereby repositioning the iliac crest in its normal position, as well as readhering the fibers of the external and internal oblique musculature to the free edge of the iliac crest.

The closed-suction drain, as stated, is placed in the iliac fossa and brought out through the corner of the fascial closure. Residual secondary fascial closure is then made between the external oblique aponeurosis immediately superior to the iliac crest closure, and this is sutured to the fascia of the gluteus maximus and tensor fascia lata. A subcutaneous closure is made through the deep level of the subcutaneous fascia, and the two-layer closure of the skin is then performed, with the drain being brought out the posterior extent of the skin incision.

The iliac bone can be used for reconstruction of up to a 4 × 4 cm defect within the calverium. Bilamellar as well as unilamellar iliac bone can be used. The advantages of unilamellar harvesting are greater stability of the iliac wing, as well as earlier ambulation. When a dual-table harvesting of the iliac is performed, patients frequently experience a 2- to 3-week period of decreased ambulation postoperatively. They often require early postoperative crutch ambulation.

The iliac bone itself, when used for a cranioplast, can be bent in a manner similar to costal bone grafts; however, it is more rigid and brittle in nature and frequently cracks on manipulation. The sole advantage of iliac bone over that of costal bone is that the cancellous bone can be packed at the junction of the cranial bone to the iliac table. Cancellous bone has a recognized superiority for early revascularization, and thereby leads to rapid incorporation of the iliac bone graft into the operative cranioplasty site.

Summary

The performance of cranioplasties using autogenous bone has a simply stated superiority: a bony defect has been reconstructed with bone. The reluctance of the neurosurgical community to attempt autogenic cranioplasties has been predicated on donor site morbidity and resorption leading to poor aesthetic results.

The hierarchy of autogenous bone reconstruction remains: (1) cranial bone, (2) costal bone, and (3) iliac bone. Cranial bone provides an extensive donor bank without a secondary donor scar distant to the operative site. The membranous nature of cranial bone provides a higher resistance to resorption and therefore provides greater assurance of lasting aesthetic results. Finally, the morbidity associated with cranial bone harvesting is the same as cranial flap elevation and thereby returns the neurosurgeon to his area of expertise.

Rib grafts are plagued by resorption problems but, similar to cranial bone grafts, have reported infection rates of 1 to 2%. Availability is limited to approximately 6 × 6 cm areas (in two ribs) and the procedure requires a second donor site.

Iliac bone grafts other than the cancellous component have no clear advantage and are therefore not recommended.

Search for the Ideal Cranioplast

The surgical archives bear witness to the surgeon's pursuit of relatively ideal cranioplastic material: everything from cadaver bones to plastic have been used. Firtell and Grisius[6] identified the attributes of the ideal material, stating that it should be: (1) inert, (2) malleable, (3) available, (4) radiolucent, (5) sterile, (6) durable, (7) nonconductive, (8) biocompatible, and (9) inexpensive.

Unfortunately, no material, other than cranial bone itself, fulfills these requirements. Metals are thermally conductive and, apart from aluminum, radiopaque. Acrylic resins and other polymers, because of their failure to incorporate bio-

Figure 3-15. An example of a poorly designed methyl methacrylate plate. Due to a rough edge and some exposed wire, this plate eroded out through the skin and became exposed in several locations. This flap was also placed under radiated scalp, which compromised the flap even further.

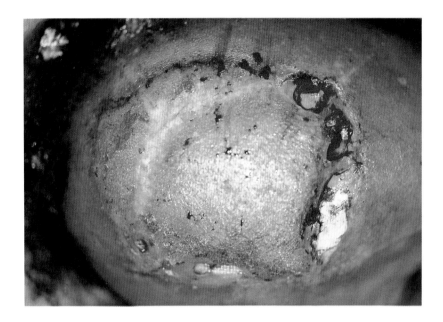

logically, remain as foreign bodies with risks of infection and exposure (Figs. 3-15, 3-16).

Despite the limitations of allogenic materials, they remain the most frequent form of cranioplastic reconstruction, favored for their availability and relative ease of molding, without subjecting the patient to donor site harvesting.

The Methyl Methacrylate Technique

Polymeric chemistry began in the 1930s and by the 1940s methyl methacrylate had been used as a cranioplast material. As use of the material spread, reports of fractures appeared in the literature, prompting Galicich and Hovind[7] to incorporate wire mesh within the methyl methacrylate.[7] The following technique is the authors' modification of their repair.

The technique for acrylic methyl methacrylate cranioplasty in the calvarium is straightforward. The donor site is prepared in the usual fashion. The bony margins must be fresh with no granuloma or fibrotic scar tissue present. The surgeon must inspect for any dural tears, which must be closed in a watertight fashion. A wire mesh template is made that can be either fitted under the bony edges or a groove can be made in the diploic table of the calvarium (Fig. 3-17).

Figure 3-16. The flap from Figure 3-15. It is easy to appreciate the open jagged edges of the wire mesh. These rough surfaces are what led to exposure of the acrylic flap.

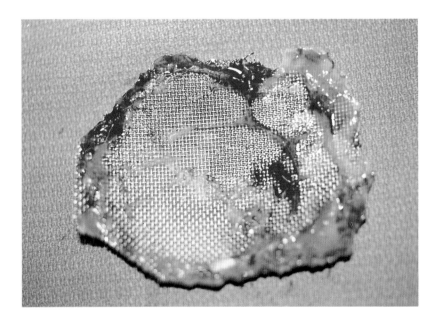

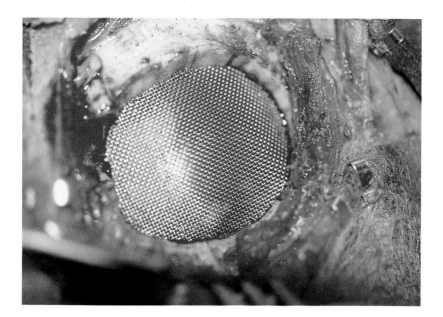

Figure 3–17.   After the craniotomy site has been prepared, the wire mesh is tucked into position with the edges carefully placed in the inner table diploic space or in the epidural space. The mesh is placed at a depth to allow at least 2 to 3 mm of acrylic to be laid over the top.

Recently, we have switched over to using titanium wire mesh for a number of reasons. Titanium is one of the best materials for biocompatibility. It is not magnetic or paramagnetic with the use of magnetic resonance imaging. Titanium is also radiolucent on plain skull x-rays and also provides for minimal artifact on computed tomography (CT). For these reasons, we have switched from stainless steel to titanium. Another important consideration is, if one is using metal, under no circumstances can one mix metals—this can and will lead to extensive corrosion and subsequent wound breakdown. This becomes particularly important in craniofacial reconstruction with the use of miniplates. The plates and screws must be of compatible metals.

In placing the wire mesh one must remember to place the mesh deep enough so that the acrylic, when laid on, does not cause an abnormally high elevation of the defect, particularly no higher than the surrounding skull. The methyl methacrylate is mixed and then applied to the wire mesh (Fig. 3–18). The consistency of

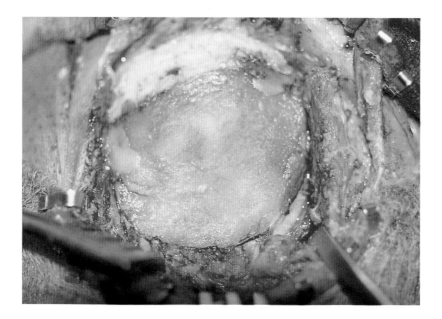

Figure 3–18.   After placement of the acrylic, the edges are checked to be sure they are smooth with no points sticking out. A high-speed round burr can be used to smooth out any high or rough spots.

the methyl methacrylate is very important. Allow it to set to a doughy or pasty thickness first. By doing this, one will prevent the runoff that can occur if it is too liquid. Remember that the methyl methacrylate is extremely exothermic, requiring a constant irrigation bath with cool saline for at least 10 to 15 minutes until the plate is totally cooled. A trick that we use is to take a piece of the methyl methacrylate, make a little ball and keep it in the hand, and as it starts to harden one can feel the exothermic reaction take place. This will allow the surgeon to gauge approximately how quickly the methyl methacrylate plate is curing. It is best to have a basin of water close by to keep one's gloves wet, and this will prevent the methyl methacrylate from sticking to the rubber gloves. One should also have available a high-speed round burr that can be used to contour the plate and level out any rough edges. A very thorough and meticulous irrigation must be done. If acrylic dust is left behind and gets into the wound, one will see Carborundum forming in the wound edges. In addition the surgeon must inspect the plate to make sure there are no rough edges, and in particular there cannot be any protruding wire mesh exposed, because these can and will erode through the skin. If the plate is wired into position, the wire edges must be turned in with no protrusion because these will also erode.

The limitations of methyl methacrylate arise from its inability to incorporate biologically; it thus acts as a foreign body surrounded by fibrous capsules. This lack of incorporation leads to the formation of sinus tracts, granulomas, erosion of the skin, and infection. Rish et al.[2] in a large series of 491 cranioplasties reported a 3.7% infection rate and a 3.1% loss of the cranioplasty. The aesthetic results of methyl methacrylate cranioplasties for small defects are favorable, but their use for large defects tends to result in contour loss.

Hydroxyapatite Cranioplast

Recent scientific advances and development of bone substitutes have led to the production of hydroxyapatite, developed by taking native coral from the sea and triphosphorylating it with high pressure in an exothermic reaction called reaminification. Following this procedure, the material's calcium triphosphate matrix resembles that of bone.[8]

The microscopic structure of hydroxyapatite is microporous, with 190 nm fenestrations, similar in size to the osteons found within native bone[9] (Fig. 3–19). This patterned porosity allows for the ingrowth of native osteocytes, and Holmes and Salyer[8] have demonstrated that as much as 30% of the volume of hydroxyapatite undergoes replacement in vivo by osteogenesis.[10]

Figure 3–19. A high-power exposure of hydroxyapatite showing the porous nature of this material with the 190 nm fenestrations. It is through these fenestrations that new bone growth occurs.

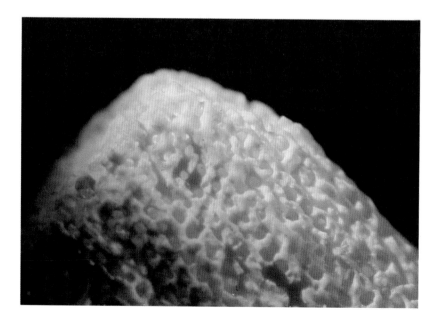

Hydroxyapatite is available as small rectangular blocks that can be contoured, using high-speed burrs, into curves and plugs suitable for defects up to 5 cm. Larger defects require special processing of the hydroxyapatite but, with three-dimensional digitization and CADCAM system milling, the Interpore ® Corporation can produce units as large as a hemi-frontal reconstruction.

After completing the contour of the hydroxyapatite with a high-speed burr, drill holes are made within the free edges of bone margin, with matching holes made within the hydroxyapatite plate. Care must be taken that a high-speed sharp drill bit is used in making the perforations within the hydroxyapatite plate, since the consistency of hydroxyapatite is much more brittle than native bone. The hydroxyapatite plate is then affixed to the surrounding bone edges, using monofilament nylon sutures. Wires are not recommended, since the process of twisting down the wires frequently fractures the hydroxyapatite.

After final fixation of the hydroxyapatite plate, the wound is irrigated with an antibiotic solution of cefazolin or bacitracin and the skull flaps replaced. A meticulous closure of soft tissues over the hydroxyapatite is necessary, since this is a foreign body, and well-vascularized soft tissue coverage is necessary to protect the artificial template from bacterial inoculation.

The advantages of hydroxyapatite are: (1) it is a prosthetic bone substitute that entails no loss of donor bone; (2) it can be fabricated preoperatively, thus saving operating time; and (3) the contouring of the hydroxyapatite is directed by CT guidance and therefore requires a minimum of surgical recontouring, thereby allowing it to be recommended for replacement of large cranial defects and also for use in cases in which extensive splitting of cranial bone has occurred. In the latter case, the hydroxyapatite is used as interposition bone substitute grafts.

The disadvantages of hydroxyapatite as a cranioplasty material are: (1) the material is a bone substitute and is therefore incompletely replaced in the osteogenesis process—only 30% of the matrix of the hydroxyapatite undergoes bony replacement, thus leading to the question of prolonged instability in its incorporated state; and (2) the material, as stated, is consider-

ably more fragile than native bone and requires greater care in handling and preparation than does autogenous bone.

Cadaveric Bone

Cadaveric bone, like hydroxyapatite, offers the operative surgeon a reconstructive option without donor site morbidity. Cadaveric bone should be considered a bone substitute, since it acts as an inert framework on which revascularization and osteogenesis can occur in a process similar to that occurring in the ossification of hydroxyapatite, while autogenous bone grafts ossify by creeping substitution of osteocytes that remain viable within the 0.2 mm bone surfaces in contact with the surrounding soft-tissue envelope.[11,12]

Currently, the only acceptable method of preserving cadaveric bone is freeze-drying. Other methods of treatment have led to denaturation of base proteins. The overwhelming problem with cadaveric bone grafts is the degree of resorption that occurs, in excess of that seen in autogenous grafts. Given the availability of other techniques, cadaveric bone grafts should be recommended only for near total cranial defects.[12]

References

1. Prolo D. Cranial defects and cranioplasty. In: Wilkins RH, Rengachary SS (eds). Neurosurgery, vol.II. New York: McGraw-Hill, 1985:1647.
2. Rish BL, Dillon JD, Meirowsky AM, et al. Cranioplasty: A review of 1030 cases of penetrating head injury. Neurosurgery 1979;4:381–5.
3. Munro IR, Guyuron B. Split rib cranioplasty. Ann Plast Surg 1981;7:341–6.
4. Zins JE, Whitaker LA. Membraneous versus endochondral bone: Implications for craniofacial reconstructions. Plast Reconstr Surg 1983;72:778.
5. Jackson IT, Munro IR, Salyer KE, Whitaker LA. Atlas of Craniomaxillofacial Surgery. St. Louis: C.V. Mosby, 1982:24–32.
6. Firtell DN, Grisius RJ. Cranioplasty of the difficult frontal region. J Prosthet Dent 1981;46:425–9.
7. Galicich JH, Hovind KH. Stainless steel mesh acrylic cranioplasty: Technical note. J Neurosurg 1967;27:376–8.
8. Holmes RE, Salyer KE. Bone regeneration in a coralline hydroxyapatite implant. Surg Forum 1978; 24:611.

9. Holmes RE. Bone regeneration with coralline hydroxyapatite implant. Plast Reconstr Surg 1979;63:626.
10. Salyer KE, Hall CD. Porous hydroxyapatite as an onlay bone graft substitute for maxillofacial surgery. Plast Reconstr Surg 1989;84:236–43.
11. Prolo DT, Burres KP, McLaughlin WT, Christensen AH. Autogenous skull cranioplasty: Fresh and preserved (frozen), with consideration of the cellular response. Neurosurgery 1979;4:18–29.
12. Abbott KH. Use of frozen cranial bone flaps for autologous and homologous grafts in cranioplasty and spinal interbody fusion. J Neurosurg 1953; 10:380–8.

F O U R

ROBERT F. KEATING, M.D.
JAMES T. GOODRICH, M.D., PH.D.

Congenital Malformations: Repair Techniques

Myelomeningocele

The treatment of myelomeningoceles, from an ethical as well as medical standpoint, has had a long and complicated history. Fortunately, the surgical approaches and techniques used today have become more consistent, as well as providing superior results both functionally and cosmetically. Currently, it is universally accepted to repair all such lesions unless an overwhelming array of other congenital anomalies predicts a dismal prognosis. Furthermore, the timing of surgery no longer generates the controversy that it once did, with the majority of defects being closed within the first 24 to 48 hours, although investigators have demonstrated no adverse effects for repairs up to 7 days.[1]

Nevertheless, there are three objectives in the repair of myelomeningoceles. The first and foremost is the need for early closure of an open cerebrospinal fluid (CSF) space. While the closure of either an open myelomeningocele or a thinly covered defect may often accelerate the course of hydrocephalus, this more importantly decreases the risk of meningitis in the newborn. A second goal paramount to the infant's future is the untethering of the newborn's spinal cord with lysis of adhesions as well as exploration and removal of any other tethering agents (i.e., hypertrophied filum, dermoid) that are occasionally found in this setting. This is undertaken to maintain whatever neurological function that exists. Finally, the role for cosmesis should not be underestimated, especially in individuals with generous defects in the underlying paravertebral skeletomuscular system.

Surgical Considerations

To appreciate fully the complexity of a myelomeningocele closure, it is vital to understand the general anatomy inherent in these defects. As seen in Figures 4-1, 4-2, 4-3, the neural placode is at or near the surface, usually covered by a thin layer of leptomeninges with the skin and subcutaneous tissue bordering circumferen-

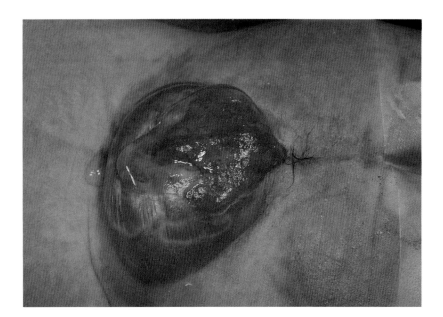

Figure 4–1. Surface view of patient with a large open lumbar myelomeningocele. The neural placode may be appreciated in the center of the lesion on the surface, as well as the presence of a CSF leak.

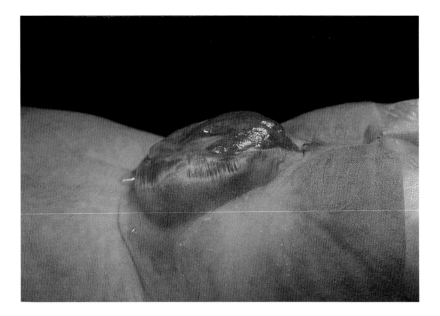

Figure 4–2. A lateral view of same patient as Figure 1 demonstrating the often elevated nature of such defects.

tially. The underlying dura is adherent to the surrounding fascia and must be eventually separated for the formation of a dural closure. Subsequently, the skin and subcutaneous tissue are employed for a full-thickness covering. In the repair of myelomeningoceles it is important to complete a five-layer closure (Table 4–1). This initially involves the isolation and tubulation of the neural placode followed by the reflection and closure of the dural remnant. Subsequently, the lumbodorsal fascia is then dissected and closed as well. It may be necessary to undermine

Table 4–1.   Myelomeningocele Repair Techniques

Five-layer closure
    Isolation and tubulation of the neural placode
    Reflection and closure of the dural remnant
    Reflection and closure of the lumbodorsal fascia
    Deep subcutaneous closure (wide undermining)
    Skin closure (avoiding edges blanching)

Figure 4–3.   A schematic illustration demonstrating the superficial nature of myelomeningoceles with their associated neural placodes. The placode is either on the surface or immediately beneath a layer of leptomeninges. Inferior to the placode is the presence of the neural roots. Great care must be taken during dissection to avoid further damage to these delicate structures.

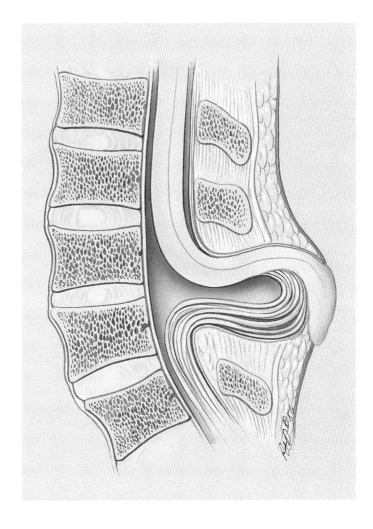

the skin widely for a deep subcuticular as well as skin closure without any detrimental tension at the skin edges.

Whereas there are an infinite variety of myelomeningocele defects, each with its own individual anatomical differences as well as surgical approaches, a few general principles apply to the majority of lesions.

Simple Myelomeningoceles

For the small to moderate-sized myelomeningocele, a transverse elliptical incision may be made around the perimeter of the lesion (Fig. 4–4). This approach was initially presented by Matson.[2] An alternative incisional approach is the use of a triangular incision around the lesion with extensions outward at the apices of the triangle. This will also yield a satisfactory closure when used with small myelomeningoceles.

Vertical skin incisions have been recommended by other authors.[3] It is thought that this affords better skin closure, being less subjected to stress from movement of the trunk musculature after surgery. Unfortunately, a vertical incision often requires a greater length, to facilitate any required undermining for closure.

Prior to the start of surgery, the myelomeningocele is protected (i.e., by doughnut) during intubation. The patient is then placed in a prone position, well cushioned on foam bolsters under the hips, ankles, and shoulders (Fig. 4–5). A three-quarter prone position can also be used for simultaneous insertion of ventriculoperitoneal shunts. Skin preparation and draping in a wide fashion is done, allowing room for a generous incision as well as for the possible eventuality of undermining adjacent subcutaneous tissues needed for satisfactory closure. Bipolar cautery is employed as well as magnification loupes.

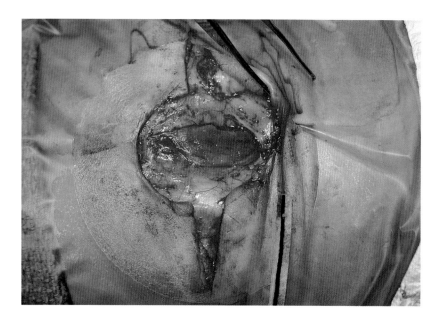

Figure 4 – 4.   Multiple approaches to the myelomeningocele repairs have been utilized. In addition to longitudinal incisions, a transverse incision offers both simplicity and sufficient exposure necessary for closing small to moderately sized myelomeningoceles. The transverse incision is centered at midposition to the defect and is extended a sufficient distance to provide room for undermining subcutaneous tissue.

After the administration of 1/4% lidocaine with 1/400,000 parts epinephrine, the incision is taken down to the level of the fascia, and using this as a plane of reference, it is then extended in both directions (away and toward the myelomeningocele) (Fig. 4 – 6). Working carefully, it is possible to define the dural neck of the myelomeningocele. The neck may then be dissected from the surrounding fascia, while observing closely for any displaced neural elements, particularly at the caudal end. It is rare that one fails to identify a dural covering and is left with a wide-open defect to close. In this setting, it may be necessary to construct a dural patch from the surrounding fascia.

If the sac has not previously been opened, it is now done in a leptomeningeal area that is thin and free of neural tissue while preserving the neural placode. The placode is dissected from the surrounding leptomeninges and epidermis (Figs. 4 – 6, 4 – 7). It is vital that all epidermoid elements are removed from the placode to avoid any later development of possible dermoid or epidermoid tumors.[4] Careful inspection is undertaken, looking for neural elements with motor rootlets being medial to the more lateral

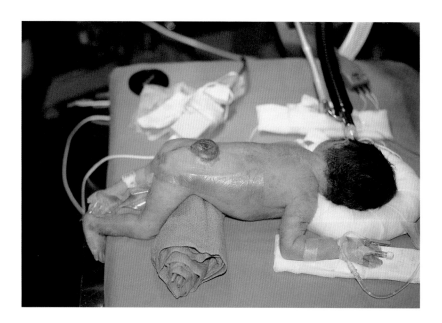

Figure 4 – 5.   The patient is positioned in a prone manner, on the end of a reversed table, so that the surgeon and assistant may sit with adequate leg room. The body is well cushioned at any pressure points (ankles, hips, shoulder, and head) with rolled towels or foam padding. In this example the patient has his ankles free over the edge of the table, with the hips supported by a rolled towel and the head by a doughnut. Notice the absence of any abdominal compression.

Figure 4–6. After generous draping (to allow extra room if needed), a transverse incision is drawn with a marking pen and then infiltrated with 1/4% lidocaine with 1/400,000 parts epinephrine. The incision is then carried away from the myelomeningocele down to the level of the paravertebral fascia. Once a plane has been established, the incision is then brought forth in the direction of the neural placode, stopping at the dural margin. After identification of the dural edge (often contiguous with the underlying fascia), dissection is then carefully continued toward the neural placode. The placode is often separated from the epidermal skin edge by a thin filament of leptomeninges. It is important to recognize this layer and to remove it with minimal manipulation of the neural placode. In addition, it is also imperative to dissect the placode completely from any surrounding epidermal tissue, whereas residual epidermis may lead to future inclusions.[4] Once the placode has been isolated, while taking care to avoid the underlying nerve roots, the neural placode is then ready for tubulation.

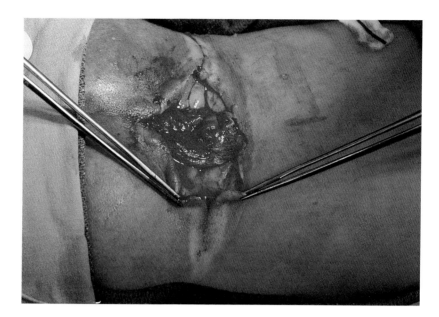

sensory roots. When the sac is empty and represents only a meningocele, it is amputated, leaving a margin for adequate closure.

The majority of myelomeningocele sacs will contain many motor and sensory elements. It is generally impossible to differentiate functional elements from atretic remnants, and thus it is imperative to assume that all tissue may be viable. These bands (neural elements) are often adherent to the wall of the sac; however, they are usually dissected easily from the dura. Excessive lifting or manipulation of the placode is to be avoided. Once dissected, the placode falls back into the canal. Should elements be inseparable from the wall of the sac, it is better to leave a portion of the wall behind.

To help reformulate the neural tube, reported to decrease the incidence of adhesions and subsequent tethering, the pial surface is closed pri-

Figure 4–7. The neural placode has been isolated and subsequently retubulated using 6-0 Prolene as a running suture through the pial membranes. This is advocated to help reduce possible intradural adhesions, which may eventually lead to tethering of the spinal cord.[5]

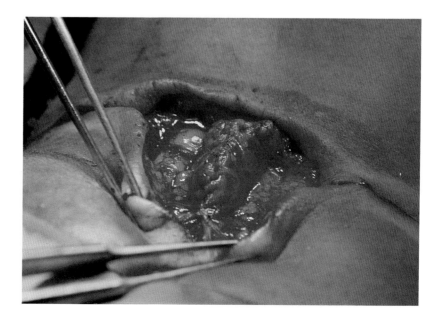

marily, as originally recommended by McLone.[5] This is done with 6-0 Prolene suture in a continuous layer. Once this is completed, the dura is then closed in a watertight fashion employing 5-0 Neurlon or any other nonabsorbable suture in a continuous layer (Figs. 4–8, 4–9).

In areas deficient of adequate material to close the neural tube in a watertight manner it may be possible to use other areas of redundant dural sac in its place. Should this prove less than satisfactory, it is often possible to substitute or reinforce the dural tube with a flap of fascia lateral to the defect and swung along its base to provide cover. It may even be necessary to rotate two flaps, one superiorly and the other inferiorly, from opposite sides to provide adequate tissue in unusually large defects. Where this proves difficult or impossible to carry out, dural substitutes utilizing silicon/Dacron grafts have been employed.[6]

Careful attention is then given with respect to the skin closure. This is paramount, especially should a dural leak develop. With small defects, this is done in two layers with interrupted absorbable sutures in the subcutaneous as well as the subcuticular layer for better cosmesis. It is important to avoid any tension on the flap, and it often is necessary to undermine the subcutaneous layer (Fig. 4–10). This is the most important layer for closure and a large majority of myelomeningoceles are easily closed primarily. When the likelihood of an incompetent dural tube exists, a running, nonabsorbable suture (i.e., 4-0 nylon) at the surface provides a more secure closure. Care must be taken to avoid too tight a skin closure to prevent any local necrosis. Areas of blanched skin may not survive, whereas dusky areas often do.

Complex Myelomeningoceles

For the exceptionally large defects (greater than 3.5 × 3.5 cm), alternative approaches have been proposed. In lesions with a very wide base it is often necessary for rotation of skin flaps at the completion of the repair. In moderately

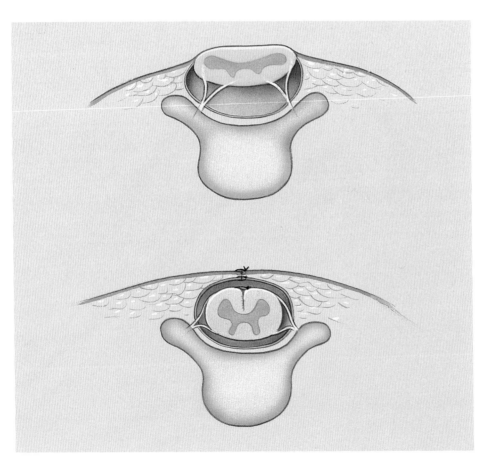

Figure 4–8. Schematic illustration demonstrating the tubulation of the neural placode as well as the dural tube. When the placode has been isolated, 6-0 Prolene suture is used, through the pial membrane to reform the spinal cord. This is done to minimize potential intradural adhesions. On completion, the dural membranes are also retubulated in a watertight fashion. The subcutaneous layers and skin are subsequently closed.

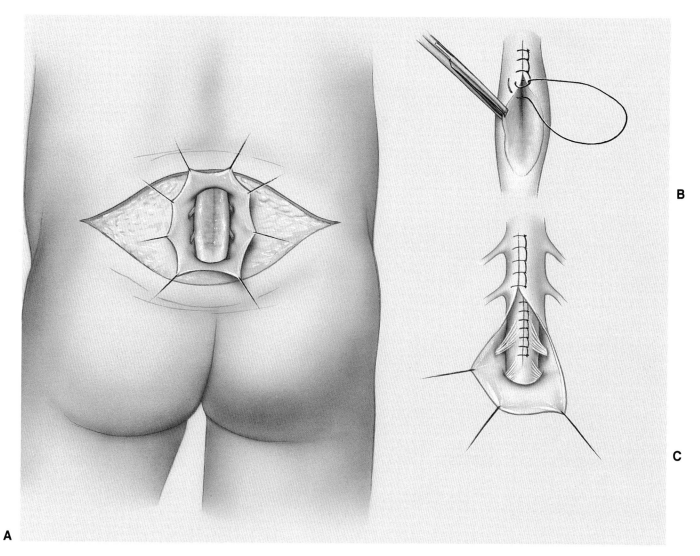

Figure 4–9. **A:** Overall view of patient after exposure of the neural placode and dural margins prior to retubulation. **B:** Demonstration of the retubulation of the neural placode using 6-0 Prolene through the pial membrane, in a running-locking stitch. Care must be taken to avoid any tension on the placode. **C:** Closure of the dural tube in a similar fashion to that used for the placode. 5-0 Neurlon (or any nonabsorbable suture) is utilized in a running-locking manner as well. It is important to close in a watertight fashion. This sometimes will require a double layer with imbrication of the dura.

sized defects this may be facilitated by the use of a standard Z-plasty technique, as seen in Figure 4–11. Alternatively, extensions of the transverse incision can be made at right angles to each end. By undermining full thickness, it is then possible to repair the defect by working from the middle of the lesion laterally.

In general, as much subcutaneous tissue as possible should be left attached to the skin. In addition, rotation flaps should have a length to base ratio of 1:1, although infants will usually tolerate 1.5:1, even across the midline.[7] In in-

fants whereby neither midline closure nor rotational pedicle flaps are possible, some authors recommend utilizing large bilateral bipedicled advancement flaps.[8] The use of myocutaneous flaps offers not only adequate thickness of skin covering but a sufficient blood supply as well, ensuring better healing at the level of skin. A particularly attractive option is the use of a Limberg-latissimus dorsi myocutaneous flap.[9] This technique employs creating a rhomboid defect over the myelomeningocele and the latissimus dorsi, along its vascular pedicle (thoracodorsal

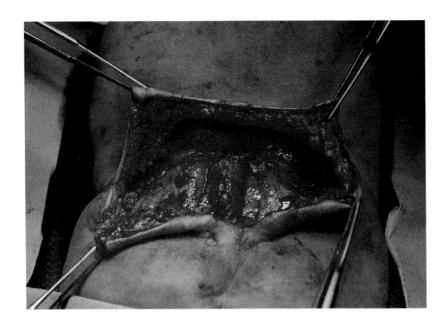

Figure 4–10. Following completion of the dural and lumbodorsal fascial closure, it is necessary to close the defect at the surface level. Depending on the size of the defect, it is generally worthwhile to undermine the subcutaneous tissue for adequate skin closure. It is important to maintain as much subcutaneous tissue underneath the skin surface as possible, to provide an adequate blood supply for healing. Care must also be taken when closing the skin edges to avoid any blanching, since these areas often fail to survive. This arterial ischemia is in contrast to dusky areas, which represent venous congestion and may remain viable. The skin is closed using a 5-0 nylon suture in a running-locking fashion.

artery) previously cut in a rhomboid shape, to fill in the defect. This technique avoids any tension on the closure as well as providing a thicker flap for protection. In addition, it is thought that the myocutaneous flap may help to prevent any kyphosis. The only disadvantage is the restriction to the thoracolumbar region. Extensive discussion on the utilization of flaps in the repair of large defects may be found in Chapter 2, "Plastic Surgery Wound Coverage for the Neurosurgery Patient."

Postoperative healing of the repair involves many variables. Perhaps the most important is the usual development of hydrocephalus. When an open myelomeningocele is closed, the course of hydrocephalus often accelerates and eventually threatens the integrity of the skin closure. Although the scope of this problem cannot be discussed at length in this chapter, it is preferable to place a ventricular shunt as early as possible in this circumstance. Chronic leakage of CSF will eventually lead to a CSF fistula as well as

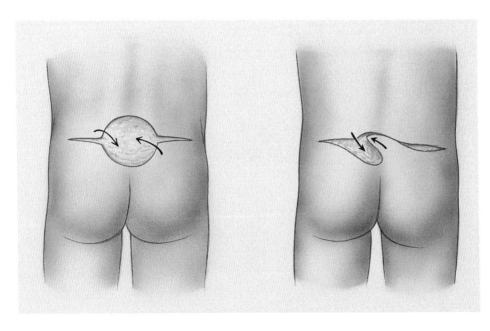

Figure 4–11. Schematic diagram representing a standard Z-plasty technique for closure of large defects. After sufficient undermining, taking care to preserve the subcutaneous layer, it is possible to advance the flap medially to cover the center of the defect overlying the dural tube. This pedicle will be able to maintain a better blood supply and thus be more likely to remain viable. Great care must be taken to avoid any skin edges from blanching.

the possibility of meningitis. In this situation, antibiotics for central nervous system coverage should be continued as long as the leak persists. Otherwise, postoperative antibiotics are continued only for 24 hours. Aside from this consideration, it is imperative to keep the patient flat, preferably head down with the buttocks up, to decrease the CSF pressure at the dural closure. In addition, the patients should be kept off their backs as well as maintaining a dry environment (without stool or urine) with the use of a waterproof plastic skirt over the buttocks/incision. Sutures are allowed to remain for 10 days or longer in the case of CSF leak.

Encephaloceles

Encephaloceles are defined as an "extracranial protrusion through a congenital opening in the skull, usually in the midline, of meninges, CSF, and/or cerebral parenchyma." The defect may contain only meninges and CSF or cerebral tissue as well. Unless one is in the Far East (Thailand, Burma, or India), encephaloceles are occipital 80% of the time, parietal 10%, and frontal 8 to 9%.[10] Regardless of the site, a few simple tenets apply to the repair of these lesions at all sites.

Preoperatively, it is important to understand and define the actual defect and whether there is the presence of any cerebral tissue contained within. With current neuroradiological technique, this is most easily evaluated by a combination of computed tomography (CT) and magnetic resonance imaging (MRI) (Figs. 4–12, 4–13). Plain skull films and tomography may also be of assistance in evaluating the bony defect, especially for those encephaloceles located in an anterior or basal location.

The objectives of surgical intervention involve replacement or removal of the extracranial tissue, closure of the dura, and repair of the bony defect with an adequate dermal covering. Encephaloceles arising from a parietal or occipital location more often may contain a significant amount of cerebral tissue, which is dependent on the size of the bony opening. Although this may often be devitalized material, such is not always easily determined preoperatively. A report by Alterman et al.[11] has demonstrated that encephaloceles may have viable tissue, although this may be of entirely glial elements. The most informative test in this instance may be an angiogram[12] to determine vascular supply to the protruding mass. In the event that the tissue is not viable, this will simplify the repair greatly. In locations where the tissue is nonfunctional, it is simply a matter of ligating the dural sac at the neck and removing the extracranial mass. This obviously may be more complicated when the superior sagittal sinus is involved (seen in Figs. 4–17, 4–18, 4–19).

Figure 4–12. Axial CT view through the nasal cavity demonstrating the presence of cerebral parenchyma within the nose, thus explaining the common occurrence of hypertelorism in these individuals. Both CT and MRI offer excellent views of the frontal base in evaluating nasofrontal encephaloceles. In this example the walls of the lateral nasal cavity are bowed out and thinned, thus representing a benign process. Coronal as well as sagittal views are often very helpful and should be included in a thorough radiologic workup of hypertelorism and a suspected nasal encephalocele.

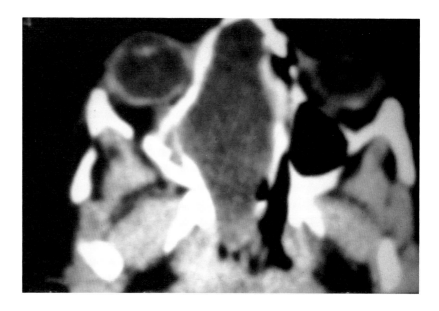

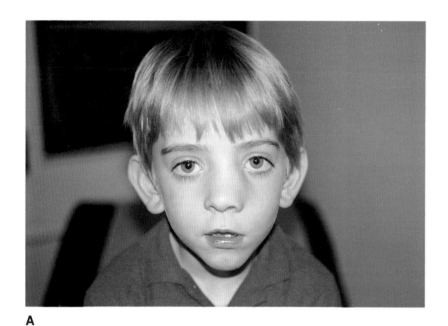

A

Figure 4–13. **A:** Photograph of a patient with a frontonasal encephalocele. Note the hypertelorism as well as the broadened nose, especially on the left. Examination of the left nares revealed a 1.5 × 1.5 cm polypoid lesion. **B:** An illustration of the patient with the nasofrontal encephalocele and associated hypertelorism. These lesions often penetrate the frontal base through the cribiform plate and may permit moderately large amounts of parenchyma to leave the intracalvarial compartment. **C:** A lateral depiction of the frontonasal encephalocele with the cribiform defect allowing significant cerebral herniation into the nasal cavity. Once the tissue is removed, from above as well as below, it is necessary to cover the defect with autologous bone.

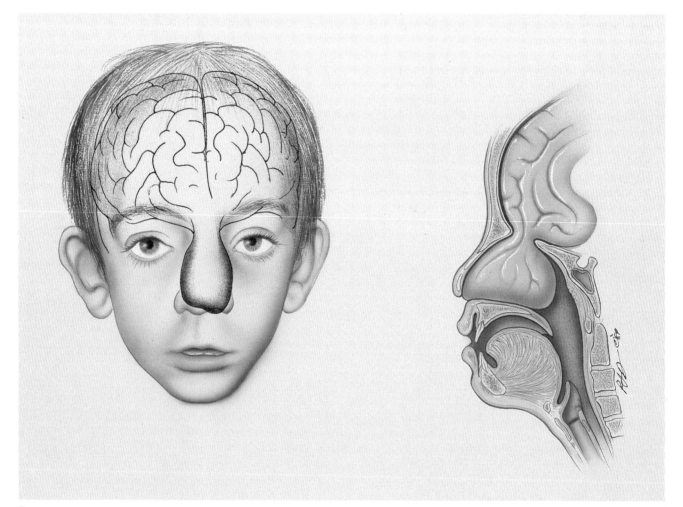

B   **C**

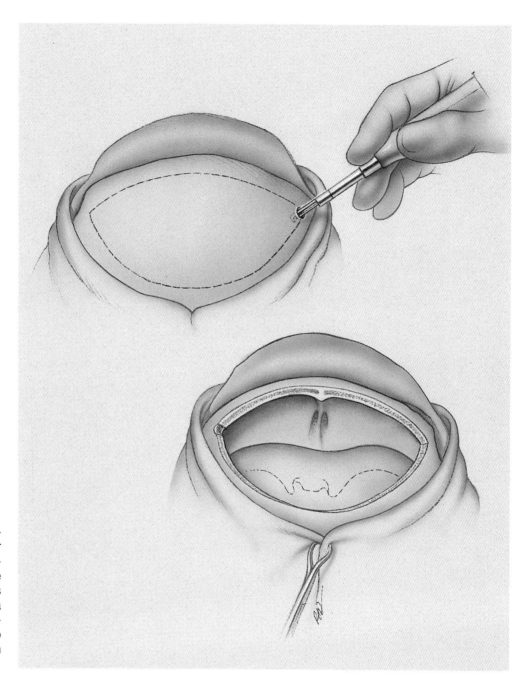

Figure 4–14. A schematic view of the anterior frontal fossa where the typical defect will lie in the cribiform plate region. It is this region that will need a repair done with a split-thickness bone graft to prevent herniation through the open space.

Although the principle of repair remains identical at all locations, it is convenient to characterize repairs located at the frontonasal, frontal, or parieto-occipital regions.

Frontonasal

Frontal and basal encephaloceles[13-15] may involve the nasofrontal, naso-orbital, or ethmoidal bones, in addition to the cribiform plate and even the superior orbital fissure (Fig. 4–13). Regardless of the site, these lesions may be reached via a standard bifrontal craniotomy for exposure of the floor of the frontal fossa. Occasionally a pterional approach may be more advantageous for encephaloceles at the temporal bone or superior orbital fissure.

The patient is placed in a supine position with the head in a neutral position but elevated 30°.

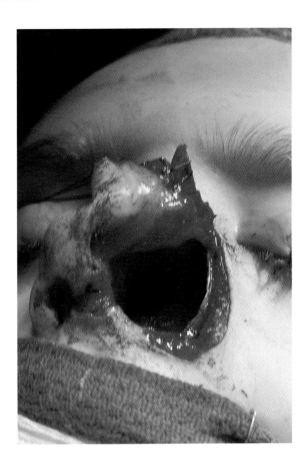

Figure 4–15.   A standard bicoronal craniotomy for an intracranial but extradural exposure is made (Fig. 4–14). With retraction of the frontal lobes, this permits identification of the bony defect in the floor (usually the cribiform plate) and allows dissection about the parenchymal stalk to free it from its bony confines. Once this has been isolated, it is then possible to ligate the stalk prior to its amputation. Demonstrated at left is the lateral rhinotomy utilized for exposure of the encephalocele from below. This is often helpful, especially for large masses. Once the encephalocele has been removed, it is necessary to reconstruct the floor of the bony defect with autologous bone (i.e., cranium). Should any dural leaks or wide-open communication with the nasal sinuses exist, it is beneficial to use pericranium (previously saved) as an intracalvarial flap.

After adequate shaving and preparation of the bifrontal area, as well as preoperative prophylactic antibiotics for staphylococcal and streptococcal coverage, 1/2% lidocaine with 1/200,000 parts epinephrine is used to infiltrate a standard bifrontal skin incision. The flap is reflected anteriorly, carefully preserving the pericranium, which is often needed subsequently for dural repair.

When undertaking the bone work, a minimal number of burr holes is made for cosmesis. This may be accomplished by a single hole adjacent to the sagittal sinus, at the superior extent of the planned bone flap. The remainder of the bone work is made with a high-speed, thin foot craniotome. In many instances, it is helpful to employ the use of a high-speed drill (e.g., Midas Rex) for the bone work. The use of this instrument offers a smaller burr hole as well as a narrower cut during the craniotomy. Furthermore, the Midas may be used to take a split-thickness graft from the inner table of the calvarium, which can subsequently be used to fill the bony defect on the floor (Figure 4–14).

It is usually necessary to repair the frontal encephaloceles intradurally. This is necessary secondary to the need to amputate the extension of tissue, followed by dural closure. In examples with nasal, pharyngeal, or sphenoidal extension, it is easier and safe to leave these extensions behind. However, encephaloceles whose mass poses problems, as in the case with a large nasal encephaloceles or orbital lesion, leading to hypertelorism, these need to be excised with a craniofacial reconstruction (see Chapters 5 and 6 for midface reconstruction techniques for hypertelorism). After defining the defect in the frontal floor, often in the region of the cribiform plate (Figs. 4–13B,C, 4–14), the cerebral hernia is dissected from the edges, leaving a dural tube that can easily be ligated with a purse string suture. Once ligated, the stalk is amputated and returned to an intracranial position.

Many examples in the literature document the need for a combined nasal and intracranial approach to large nasoethmoidal encephaloceles.[14,15] This facilitates the removal of the nasal mass and may even allow the intracranial work to proceed extradurally (Fig. 4–14, 4–15). Regardless of the location, it is imperative that repairs be watertight, especially with the presence of the nearby sinuses. Should primary repair be impossible or difficult, as it can be in this location, the pericranium previously preserved and protected can now be employed to provide a dural graft. Other materials (i.e., fascia lata, temporalis fascia, etc.) may also be used here.

The bony defect must be repaired to prevent brain herniation, and it is recommended that autologous bone be used when possible, especially with the proximity of the sinuses precluding any desire to use a foreign body. It is often easy to remove a diploic portion of the inner table of the skull (from the bone flap) to fashion a repair (discussed in Chapter 3). The overlying dura will epithelialize well over the autologous bone.

The incision is closed in a routine manner, while employing a subgaleal drain. Prophylactic antibiotics are routinely maintained postoperatively for 24 hours, unless communication exists between the CSF compartment and nasal area. In this case they are continued for 7 days.

Parieto-Occipital

The more common lesion found in the parieto-occipital region requires the same objective for successful repair. It is important to isolate the herniated cerebral tissue to remove or reduce and to follow this with closure of the bony defect. The viability of the underlying tissue can be examined preoperatively with physical studies (i.e., visual evoked potentials,[16] positron emission tomography, brain scan). This may be of assistance in examples whereby it is difficult to determine if the herniated tissue is necrotic. Prior tissue culture studies have demonstrated that this tissue may only represent glial tissue.[11] Obviously, it is desirable to leave functional cerebral tissue intact and within the patient. Tissue that has necrotic features should be amputated (Figs. 4–16–4–20). For lesions lying over the midline, it is necessary to evaluate the status and location of the major venous structures (i.e., superior sagittal sinus). It is recommended that one be cognizant of the presence of the sinus preoperatively rather than in the operating theater. Should the sinus be encountered, its preservation is most often required (in examples of posterior lesions).

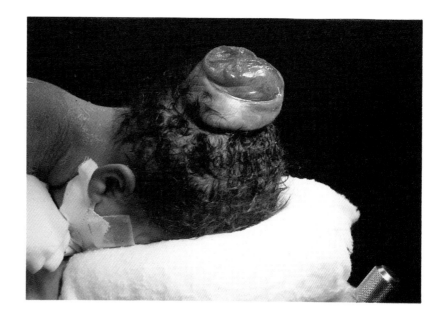

Figure 4–16. This child had a large midline occipital encephalocele. Preoperatively, the superior sagittal sinus appeared to be patent, thus complicating the repair. Nevertheless, the patient is placed in a prone position with the head supported by a well-padded cerebellar head-rest. A generous shave and preparation is then instituted before incision is made.

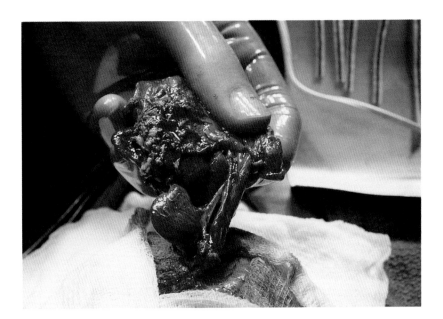

Figure 4–17. After having made an elliptical skin incision about the base of the encephalocele, and dissecting the dural edges from the parenchyma, one is left with the herniation sac. In this example the sinus was open and thus had to be dissected free from the surrounding tissue. The remainder of tissue is then amputated carefully. A watertight dural closure is essential, using pericranium or other substitute if necessary. Subsequently, the bony defect must be closed. This is most easily facilitated by using the inner table of the skull from an adjacent area (via the Midas Rex). Skin closure, utilizing a subgaleal and cutaneous layer, may require trimming excess skin edges for a satisfactory result.

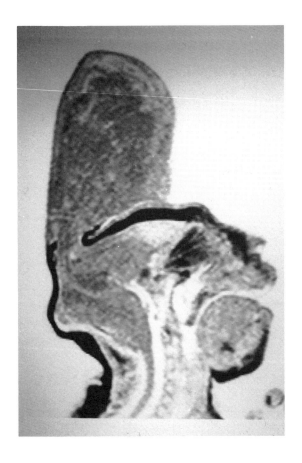

Figure 4–18. An MRI of a severe anencephalic with a significant occipital encephalocele. Note the bony defect in the midline with hindbrain structures being present but minimal cerebral cortex. In this example all of the herniated tissue was gliotic as demonstrated by tissue culture.

The patient is positioned in a prone manner and is supported by a padded cerebellar head-rest (Fig. 4 – 19). It is vital that the eyes, nose, and mouth are well protected. A transverse elliptical skin incision is usually made to provide adequate skin closure. Once the pericranium is identified and carefully separated from the contents of the herniated sac, the encephalocele is simply amputated (Figs. 4 – 17, 4 – 20). Subse-quently, after the lesion is excised, the dura should be closed in a watertight fashion, utilizing a patch graft if necessary. At this time, it is helpful to have assessed the true extent of the bony defect preoperatively. In older children, the defect is handled in a similar manner to that for anterior lesions, previously discussed in this chapter. Infants, however, require a delayed repair of the calvarium in view of their growth and

Figure 4 – 19. An anencephalic patient (as seen in Figure 4 – 18) in position for repair. The patient is supine at 30° with the head supported by a well-padded cerebellar head-rest, allowing the encephalocele to hang freely.

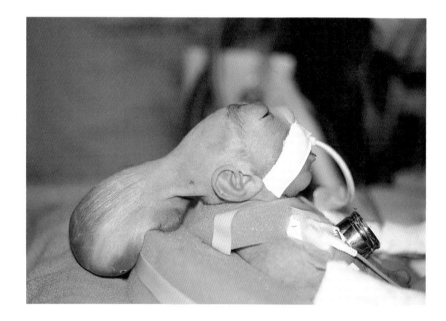

Figure 4 – 20. After making transverse incisions to the encephalocele sac, the pericranium is identified and separated from the dura. The cerebral stalk is then isolated as well as the sinus. In this case the sinus was nonfunctioning, and the herniated sac was simply amputated. However, in patients with a patent sinus it is clear that this should be preserved in this posterior setting. In this case, the sinus must carefully be dissected from the surrounding tissue. Following the removal of the encephalocele, it is also imperative to ensure a watertight dural closure. Bony repair in an infant has often been delayed, although we now place a piece of bone from an adjacent area of the skull in the region of the defect. This will often grow and fill in the defect if it is in the presence of the pericranium or periosteum. Skin closure is completed with a 4-0 nylon suture in a running-locking stitch.

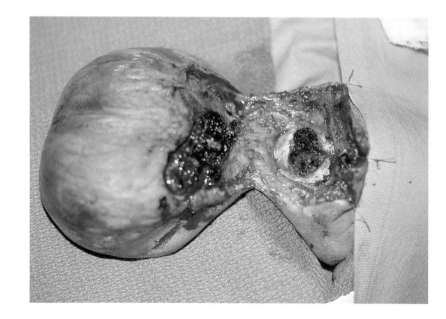

lack of a diploic table. We have, however, occasionally taken a piece of adjacent bone and grafted this into the affected area and found this to fill in over time.

Frequently, the bony defects may be extensive, which may require more bone than the autologous grafts (calvarium, ribs, etc.) can provide (Fig. 4–21). Here it may be necessary to delay reconstruction. Nevertheless, after excising the encephaloceles, redundant skin is invariably present. It is a simple matter to remove this, being careful to allow ample skin to avoid any tension on the incision. We routinely use a subgaleal drain to minimize postoperative collections. Consequently, we continue the use of antibiotics for 24 hours after removal of the drain.

Those with anterior defects and encephaloceles have a much better prognosis[17] secondary to less brain being herniated. The majority of these children lead normal lives if no other congenital defects are present. On the other hand, posterior encephaloceles have a much poorer outcome. Only 20 to 30% have normal intellect, and this is further complicated by a 50% association with hydrocephalus and its attendant problems.

Human Tails

Although true human vestigial tails may be an uncommon occurrence, literature does report such examples,[18-21] and one occasionally encounters such a rarity. By definition a "true tail" may contain adipose, connective tissue, striated muscle, blood vessels, nerves, all covered by skin (Fig. 4–22). Bone, spinal cord, cartilage, and notochord are lacking. This is in contrast to "pseudotails," which represent a more variable lesion, encompassing teratomas, lipomas, prolongation of coccygeal vertebrae, myelomeningoceles, and other miscellaneous tumors (Fig. 4–23B).

An additional differentiating feature is the superficial nature of true tails. These appendages are generally limited by the paravertebral fascia and thus their repair is facilitated versus the more complicated and varied surgical intervention necessary for pseudotails. It is imperative that one evaluate the underlying neural tube in these cases, demonstrating any communication between neural elements and the surface (Fig. 4–24). This is easily done with CT or MRI today (Fig. 4–23A).

Nevertheless, for simple true tails the surgical approach is similar to that taken for the myelo-

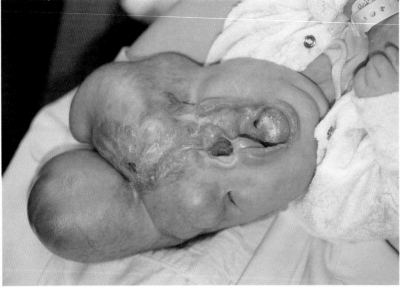

A

Figure 4–21. **A:** A complicated holo cranial encephalocele involving the midface with clefting and the entire calvarium. In this child there was no development of the calvarium with complete lack of bone from the ears up. The reconstruction involved not only dissection of the encephaloceles, but also a rebuilding of the calvarial vault using a combination of rib grafting and hydroxyapatite. A preoperative angiogram localized the important vascular structures, including the sagittal sinus, which is between the two large superior encephaloceles. *(Figure Continues.)*

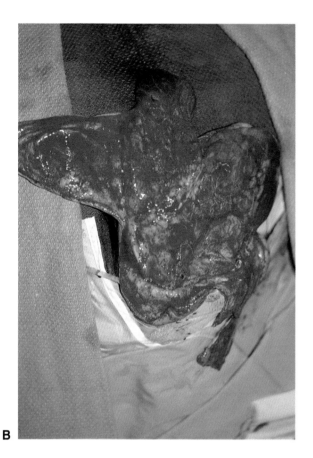

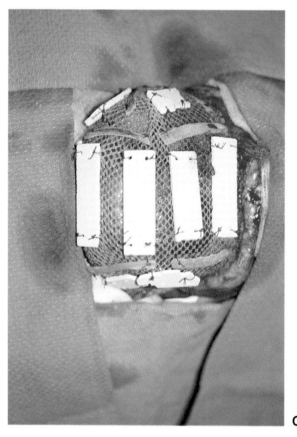

B

C

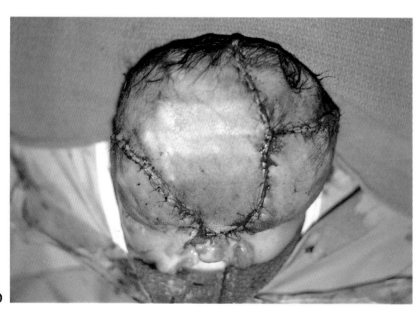

D

Figure 4 – 21 *(continued).* **B:** The dissection of the encephaloceles is completed, allowing for generous full-thickness skin to cover the repair site. In this case the dissection had to be carried down to expose the normal bone rim. **C:** A Dacron mesh graft was first fashioned to make a template for the calvarium. Using split rib grafts from the patient and hydroxyapatite (see Chapter 3 for a full discussion of these techniques), a matrix was built to provide a new calvarium. **D:** An intraoperative photograph showing the calvarium reconstruction with the remodelled flaps back in position. At a six-month interval the patient can then be brought back for a midface monobloc clefting repair once the calvarial grafts have taken.

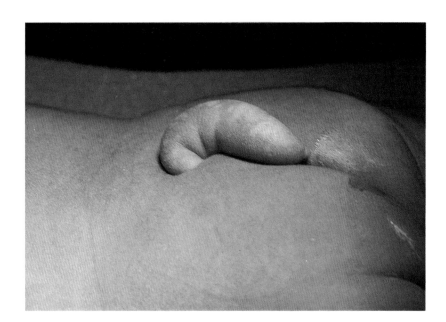

Figure 4–22.   An example of a human tail. This lesion was midline and was composed entirely of adipose and connective tissue without any apparent subfascial communication to underlying neural structures. However, on closer scrutiny, the MRI (Fig. 4–23A) demonstrated an underlying lipoma.

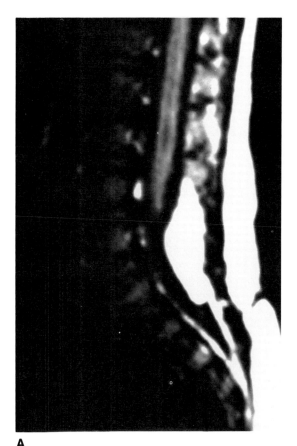

A

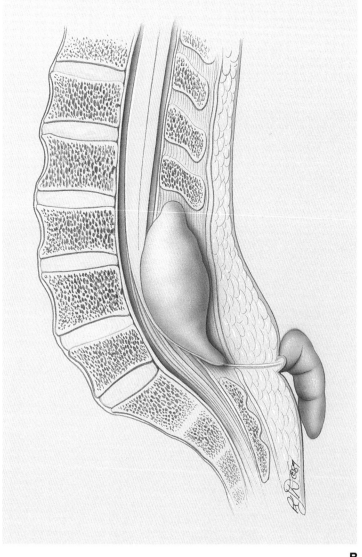

Figure 4–23.   **A:** An MRI demonstrating the presence of a dermal sinus tract communicating with an underlying lipoma. This is illustrated schematically in **B**. While true tails are defined as superficial lesions only, pseudotails may mimic this entity, but may have a complex underlying structure (i.e., lipoma, dermoid, teratoma, etc.). It is thus crucial to rule out any deep associated lesions with tails. This can easily be accomplished today with the use of MRI.

B

Figure 4–24. An intraoperative photograph showing a fibrous stalk in the center of the dissection along with a defect in the lumbodorsal fascia. Should any dermal sinus tract be discovered, it is then followed inferiorly to its termination. These sinus tracts will often lead to lipomas or other tumors and thus it is important to be thorough. It may be appreciated here that there is a defect in the fascia, thus raising suspicion to an underlying process. In the case of a simple or superficial tail, once its origin at the paravertebral fascia is identified, it is simply amputated at the base. The skin incision is then closed in a routine fashion.

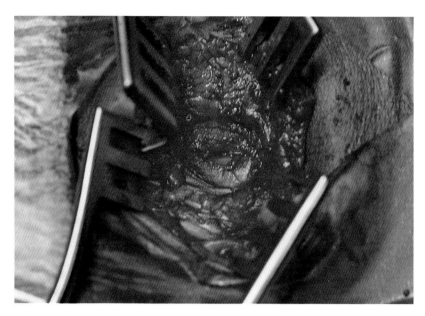

meningocele. The child is placed in the prone position on bolsters, with a generous area prepared and draped for excision of the tail. After administration of prophylactic antibiotics, a transverse incision is made circumferentially around the dermal appendage. The subcutaneous layer is dissected carefully, preserving any fibrous stalk that is often present. It is important to follow this stalk; should it cross the paravertebral fascia, this would indicate a more complicated lesion (Fig. 4–24). After confirming that the dermal appendage does indeed terminate at the fascia, it is simply amputated. Closure is simple with a layer of absorbable sutures in the subcutaneous layer and either another absorbable layer in the subcuticular layer or nonabsorbable suture through the surface. Depending on the original size of the tail, it may be necessary to trim some of the incisional edge to provide a better elliptical closure.

Postoperative wound care is straightforward, with sutures being removed 10 days later. It is important to keep the area clean and dry from the infant's urine and stool. This can be facilitated by the use of a plastic skirt below the lesion covering the buttocks.

References

1. Charney EB, Weller SC, Sutton LN, et al. Management of the newborn with a myelomeningocele: Time for a decision-making process. Pediatrics 1985;75:58.
2. Matson DD. Neurosurgery of infancy and childhood, 2nd ed. Springfield IL: Charles C Thomas, 1969.
3. Bannister C. A method of repair of myelomeningocele. Br J Surg 1972;59:6.
4. Martinez-Lage JF, Masegosa J, Sola J, et al. Epider-
moid cyst occurring within a lumbosacral myelomeningocele. J Neurosurg 1983;59:1095.
5. McLone DG. Technique for closure of a myelomeningocele. Childs Brain 1980;6:65.
6. Bartal A, Heilbronn Y, Plashkes Y. Reconstruction of the dural canal in myelomeningocele. Plast Reconstr Surg 1970;47:1.
7. Davies D, Adendorff DJ. A large rotation flap raised across the midline to close a lumbosacral myelomeningocele. Br J Plast Surg 1977;30:166.
8. Zook E, Dzenitis A, Bennet J. Repair of a large myelomeningocele. Ann Surg 1969;98:41.
9. Munro R, Neu BR, Humphreys RP. Limberg-latissimus dorsi myocutaneous flap for closure of myelomeningoceles. Childs Brain 1983;10:381.
10. Ingrahm FD, Matson DD. Neurosurgery of infancy and childhood. Springfield, IL: Charles C Thomas, 1954.
11. Alterman RA, Goodrich JT, Morrison RM, Moskal JR. Primary encephalocele cultures can yield pure populations of normal human astrocytes. In press.
12. Gilmore RL, Kalsbeck JE, Goodman JM, et al. Angiographic assessment of occipital encephaloceles. Radiology 1972;103:127.
13. Suwanella C, Hongsaprabhas C. Frontoethoidal encephalomeningocele. J Neurosurg 1966;25:172.
14. Griffith BH. Frontonasal tumors: Their diagnosis and management. Plast Reconstr Surg 1976;57:692.
15. Luyendijk W. Intranasal encephaloceles: A survey of 8 neurosurgically treated cases. Psychiatr Neurol Neurochir 1969;72:77.
16. Engel R, Buchan GC. Occipital encephaloceles with and without visual evoked potentials. Arch Neurol 1974;30:314.
17. Mealy J Jr, Dzenitis AJ, Hockey AA. Prognosis of encephaloceles. J Neurosurg 1970;32:309.
18. Dao AH, Netsky MG. Human tails and pseudotails. Hum Pathol 1984;15:449.
19. Spiegelmann R, Schinder E, Mordejai M, Blakstein A. The human tail: A benign stigma. J Neurosurg 1985;63:461.
20. Ledley FD. Evolution and the human tail: A case report. N Engl J Med 1982;306:1212.
21. Keating RF, Goodrich JT. A tale of two tails. In preparation.

FIVE

JAMES T. GOODRICH, M.D., PH.D.

Craniofacial Reconstruction for Craniosynostosis

This chapter will deal with some of the recent surgical techniques that have been developed for treatment of congenital craniofacial disorders. The emphasis will be strictly on the surgical techniques and not on the developmental or etiologic problems associated with congenital craniosynostosis.

The history of surgery in craniofacial disorders goes back many years. From an anatomic point of view, the appreciation of suture dysfunction and premature synostosis dates at least to the early part of the 16th century. In the work of Hundt[1] is evidence that an early anatomist appreciated the suture patterns that could occur in any of a number of different configurations. Dryander,[2] in 1537, illustrated some excellent examples of suture fusion and abnormal variations in the coronal and sagittal suture lines. Andreas Vesalius,[3] in 1543, showed a number of excellent examples of misshapen and malformed skulls: examples of oxycephaly and brachycephaly stand out in this work. In the same century, 1583, in the work of the great Italian Croce,[4] a number of examples of unusual head shapes appeared. One of the anatomic plates looks very much like a Tessier series of today. In Croce's book are examples of coronal synostosis, and even what looks like a case of Crouzon's disease is nicely outlined.

As to the surgical techniques and intervention in the treatment of synostosis, it was really not until the 19th century that surgeons began to appreciate that premature fusion could lead to maldevelopment of the brain and even in some cases microcephaly. One of the best examples of this appeared in the mid-19th century when a Frenchman, Lannelungue,[5,6] performed a craniectomy for treatment of a child with microcephaly. By the later half of the 19th century, there were already a number of excellent surgical textbooks appearing, showing different techniques for treatment of premature suture fusion.[7-9] In 1895 Dennis[7] published a number of figures showing various types of synostectomies being performed for the treatment of premature fusion. In San Francisco by 1896, a Dr. L. C. Lane[8] had published one of the first American surgical interventions for craniosynostosis.

Dr. Lane presented a classic case of a mother who came into his office and gave the following plea: "My child's brain is locked up and can you unlock it"? Dr. Lane described a 15-month-old microcephalic who "evinced few signs of mentality." He noted that the sutures were firmly ossified and recommended synostectomies, which were subsequently done. Unfortunately, the child died of anesthetic complications, but this case is certainly one of the earliest American examples.

In Scotland, William MacEwen,[9] was already introducing the morcellation technique for malshaped heads. In his book on *The Growth of Bone*, he has an excellent example of a child in whom a subtemporal and pterional morcellation was done for premature fusion. Even 80 to 100 years ago, the techniques that are still commonly used by surgeons today were available for the treatment of craniosynostosis.

The technique commonly used by neurosurgeons now, the simple craniosynostectomy, was introduced by Don Matson, Frank Ingraham, and Eben Alexander in the late 1940s.[10] The technique has been popularized in pediatric neurosurgery textbooks and still remains the most common form of treatment today.[11,12] However, with the recent introduction of craniofacial techniques, particularly from our French colleagues Paul Tessier, Daniel Marchac, D. Renier, and others, more sophisticated techniques have been adopted.[13-17] This chapter will review some of the procedures that are now being commonly used in the various craniofacial centers.

Plagiocephaly (Unilateral Coronal Synostosis)

One of the most common craniofacial abnormalities is plagiocephaly (unilateral coronal synostosis). Plagiocephaly is easily recognizable and has a number of characteristics that must be appreciated. Without an adequate appreciation of these abnormalities, the surgical treatment of this entity cannot be addressed. It is easy to understand why the older technique of just a simple coronal suture synostectomy did not lead to the resolution of the developmental anomalies that subsequently occur in plagiocephaly. When evaluating a child with plagiocephaly, one can easily appreciate the uneven orbital rim line (Figs. 5–1, 5–2). As a result of the coronal suture fusion, the child develops a flattening on one side and then a compensatory frontal bossing on the opposite forehead. There is a typical flattening of the orbital rim on the side of the synostosis and a bulging of the contralateral orbital rim. If the severity of the syndrome is significant enough, there is a complete deviation of the nasoethmoidal complex. Treatment of this disorder requires a complete disassembly of the forehead and orbital rim unit with an advance-

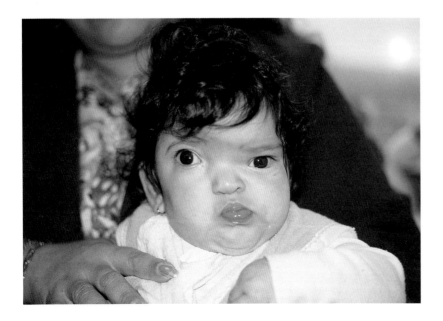

Figure 5–1. A 2-month-old child with severe plagiocephaly. Due to fusion of the child's right coronal suture, there has developed a severe left-sided compensatory frontal boss. The left orbit has been moved forward and downward. There is also significant deviation of the nasoethmoidal complex.

Figure 5–2. **A, B:** Schematic of the child in Figure 5–1 showing graphically the severe deformity that occurs in the frontal fossa. An appreciation of the sphenoid wing deviation is evident here in **A**. **B:** The degree of advancement necessary to correct this severe plagiocephaly is shown.

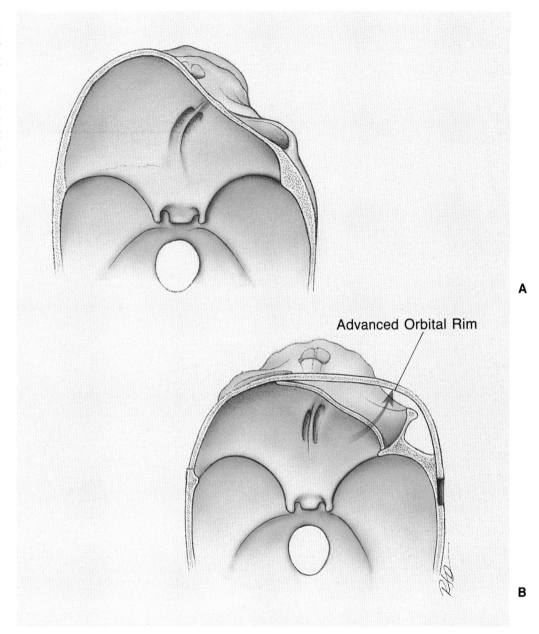

A

Advanced Orbital Rim

B

ment of the orbital bandeau, and a subsequent reconstruction of the forehead (Fig. 5–3). These surgical techniques will be gone into in some detail.

In the younger child with a unilateral coronal synostosis (Fig. 5–4), some people have advocated doing just a unilateral approach when there is not significant compensatory bossing on the opposite side. This involves doing nothing more than isolating out the orbital rim itself after doing a sectional unilateral craniotomy. As can be seen in Figures 5–5, 5–6, the surgeon first

removes a segment of forehead bone, in this case labeled B. The orbital unit is elevated from the nasal suture line, across the orbital rim, and through the zygoma. This unit is then advanced out in a tongue-in-groove fashion, and can give adequate correction via a unilateral approach (Figures 5–6, 5–7). The problems with this technique though occur as the child grows, for the development tends to remain unequal on both sides. As the child gets older, a further asymmetrical deformation can occur, particularly in adolescence. As a result of this asymmetrical

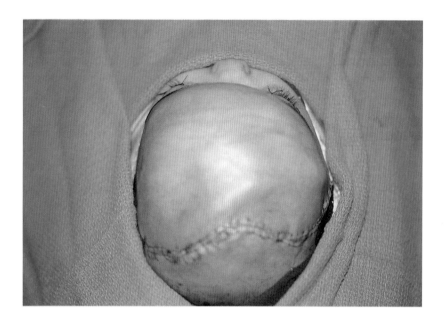

Figure 5–3. The child in Figure 5–1 after a full orbital bandeau and forehead advancement showing the symmetry expected in this type of case. This advancement corresponds to Figure 5–2B.

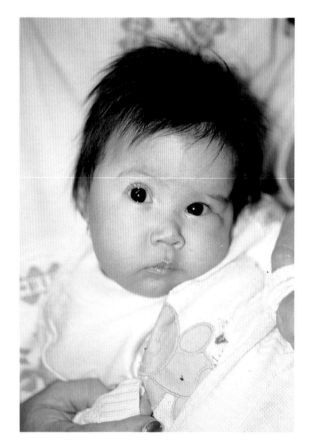

Figure 5–4. A 3-month-old child with a milder form of plagiocephaly. In this case the right coronal suture is fused prematurely, giving a left frontal compensatory boss. The orbital deviation is not as severe as in the case in Figure 5–1.

growth, most craniofacial surgeons are now using a bilateral full forehead and orbital bandeau advancement.

In Figures 5–8, 5–9, 5–10 are illustrated examples of a forehead advancement using the original orbital bandeau and then a forehead advancement technique. The surgery begins with a bifrontal coronal skin flap. A craniotomy is done removing the plate marked A in Figure 5–8. The bifrontal flap is dissected down below both orbital rims and laterally until both zygomas are exposed and the nasal suture medially. Following the cuts that are made on the segment labeled B, this bandeau is then freed and removed. This unit is now advanced forward and placed in position to correct the unilateral plagiocephaly (Figs. 5–9, 5–10). This technique is extremely useful when there is no marked deformity of the orbital bandeau itself.

Using the typical tongue-in-groove technique, a surgeon can develop from 1 to 3 cm of orbital advancement. Using wires or miniplates, the orbital bandeau is put back into position, allowing for symmetrical alignment. The forehead piece is then put back into position and either allowed to float or wired back into position. In cases where there is a sloping forehead, we have adopted a technique that was introduced by Marchac using again a tongue-in-groove technique up over the frontal boss.[15] In

Figure 5–5. **A, B:** An anterioposterior plus tilt view of a child with unilateral plagiocephaly. In this technique only one side is corrected **(A).** A craniotomy is done to elevate the bone segment labeled "B." Once this unit is removed, the surgeon can retract the frontal and temporal tips, giving good exposure of the anterior fossa. The bifrontal skin flap has to be carried down to the nasal suture medially and the zygoma laterally. The orbital rim/bandeau, here labeled "C," is removed as a unit and advanced forward. This is graphically demonstrated in Figure 5–6b.

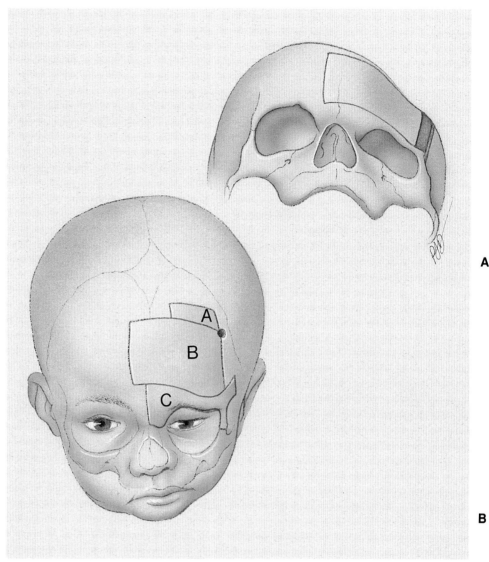

A

B

this case, a triangular pattern is cut out of the bone just behind the coronal suture (Fig. 5–11). This unit is then advanced forward and secured in place. This can allow up to 1 to 1.5 cm of forehead advancement to correct frontal flattening.

In cases in which the forehead and orbital line are severely malaligned or in the case of an older child where the bone is too thick for easy malleability, a useful technique is to make a new forehead using a section of bone from the convexity (Fig. 5–12). In Figure 5–13 is an example of a metal template that is used to mark out the calvarium area of bone that most reasonably approximates a normal forehead. Using a Marchac forehead template, a piece of the calvarium that closely approximates a normal forehead is marked out. Using these techniques, the orbital rim is removed as a unit to be replaced in an advanced position. The new forehead unit, which has been constructed from the calvarial bone, is placed back into position (Fig. 5–14). A tongue-in-groove type advancement can be done as shown in Figure 5–15. In cases in which the orbital bandeau is too deformed, this unit can also be discarded and a new unit developed from the forehead; this technique is discussed further in the section on trigonocephaly.

The orbital bandeau and forehead bones are put back into position; the remaining pieces of

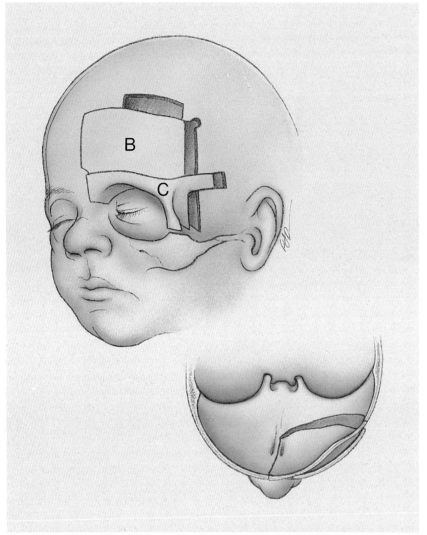

A

B

Figure 5–6.   **A, B:** A more oblique view showing the unilateral advancement after moving the orbital bandeau forward **(A).** The frontal fossa osteotomy is made in the orbital roof, as shown in **B.**

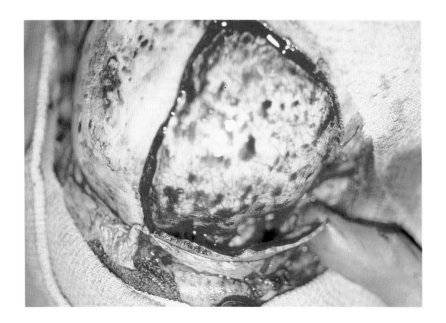

Figure 5–7.   An intraoperative view duplicating the view in Figure 5–6. The surgeon's finger is holding the orbital bandeau in the advanced position where it will be either wired or miniplated into position.

Figure 5-8. **A, B:** A schematic showing the osteotomy cuts made in a full forehead advancement. After a bicoronal skin flap is turned, the craniotomy is performed to remove the segment labeled "A" in **A.** The orbital bandeau is then removed as a unit following the cuts in the part labeled "B." **B:** A lateral projection and the cuts carried into the squamosal bone and zygoma are shown.

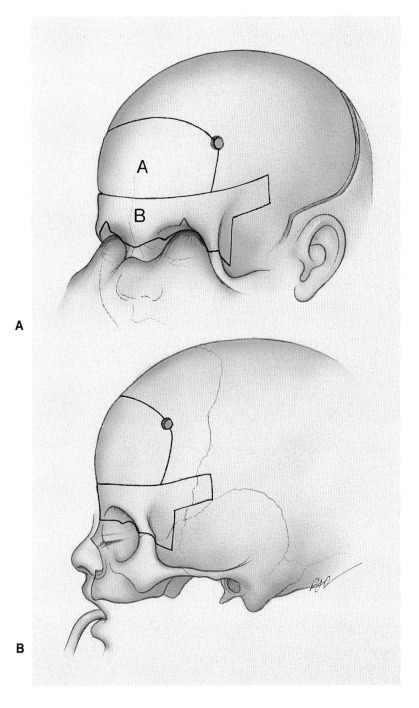

A

B

bone are put back together in a mosaic. It has been our experience that any bony defect should not be much larger than about 2 cm, because these tend not to fill in. It is very important to save the pericranial layer, and to lay that back down into position over where the craniectomies have been done. We have found that if the apex portion of the calvarium is left opened, this area tends to fill in with bone the least. As a result, we like to keep the bony defects to the lateral aspects of the skull. This will prevent a coning effect in which the brain tends to take the path of least resistance and will grow out the top of the head giving a turricephalic appearance. This type of cosmetic result is undesirable, and the easiest way to compensate for it is to allow lateral growth, which cosmetically is more appropriate.

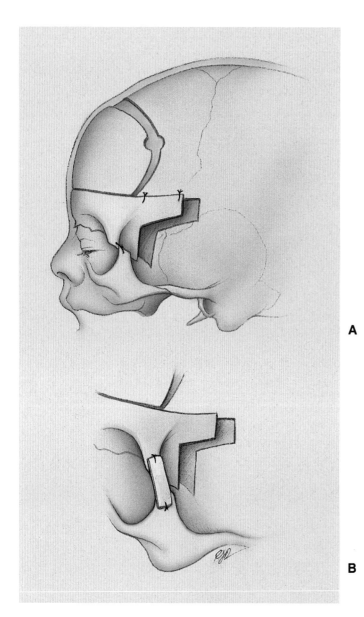

Figure 5–9. **A, B:** A schematic showing a lateral projection with the units in advanced position. **B:** The tongue-in-groove technique is shown with a bone graft over the zygomatic defect that will occur in the advancement. This piece can be easily harvested from the calvarial bone.

A

B

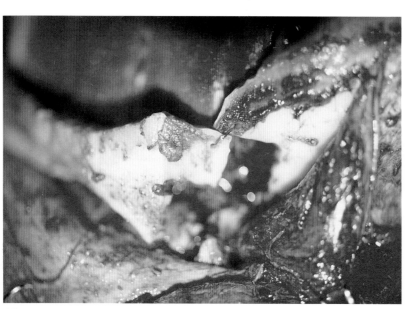

Figure 5–10. Intraoperative view showing the equivalent view of Figure 5–9B with the advancement in position. A full 15 mm advancement has been obtained in the procedure.

Figure 5–11. **A, B:** A useful technique demonstrated here showing a triangular tongue-in-groove technique where the forehead can be advanced and held in position. The triangular cuts are made just behind the coronal sutures and kept as part of the forehead flap. As the flap is replaced into an advanced position, these triangular pieces are wired "forward," as in **B.** This technique can be coupled with a full midface advancement, as shown here (and discussed further by Dr. Argamaso in Chapter 6. See also Figure 5–17.)

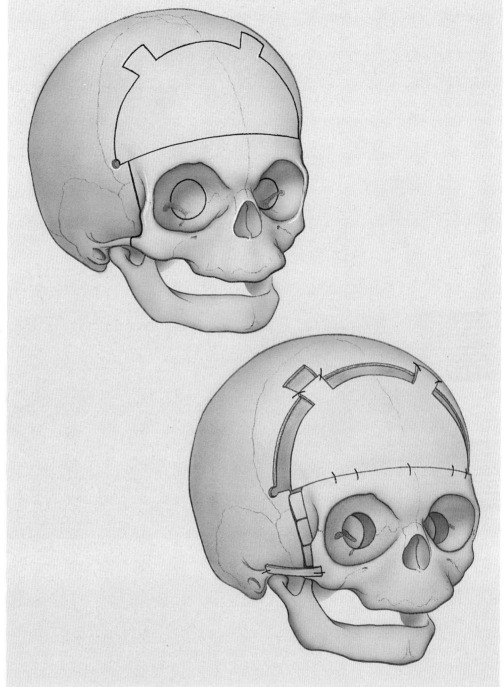

A

B

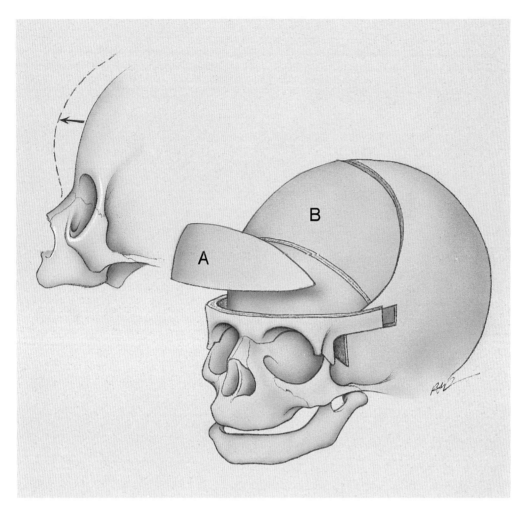

Figure 5-12. In the case of a child with severe plagiocephaly where the forehead is too deformed to use, a new forehead can be created from a higher portion of the calvarium. As diagrammatically illustrated here, two craniotomy cuts are made as outlined in parts "A" and "B." Part "B" is designed from a template, as shown in Figure 13. The orbital bandeau is elevated, as shown in the osteotomy cuts and advanced. Plate "B" will then be switched with "A" to make a new forehead (see Figure 5-15).

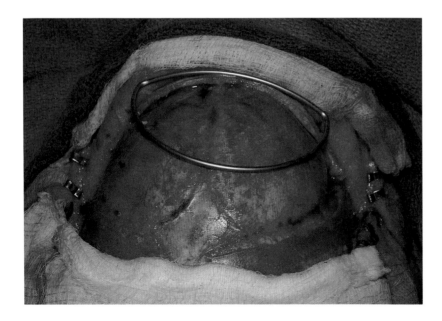

Figure 5-13. Intraoperative view with the forehead exposed after a bicoronal skin flap. Using a template, a portion of the convexity is marked out and this will be used as the new forehead unit (Figure 5-12, plate "B").

Figure 5–14. The orbital bandeau has been removed as a unit. The forehead piece has also been removed (the metopic suture was split in this child, hence the two pieces). The surgeon can then wire these pieces together as a unit to be replaced in an advanced position.

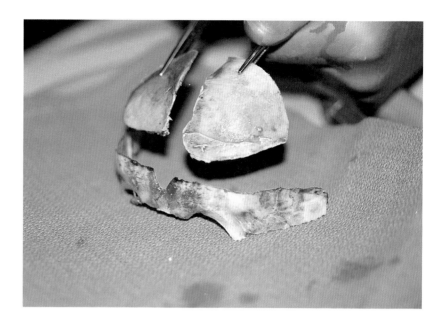

Figure 5–15. A, B: A schematic showing the orbital bandeau and forehead unit wired back in position. In some cases the piece labeled "A" goes back in segments as a mosaic to provide a good contour. **B:** A typical "tongue-in-groove" advancement is shown.

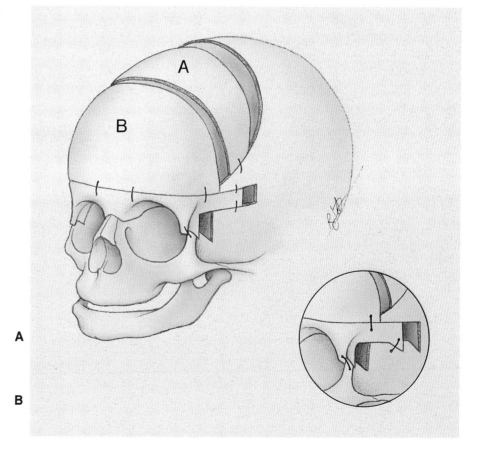

A

B

A useful additional technique that can be helpful in a case of marked frontal bossing is a dural plication. This will reduce the prominent boss and thereby provide a better contour for the overlying bone (Fig. 5–16). In a dural plication keep the sutures as superficial as possible so that there is no underlying injury to the brain. This technique can reduce a prominent boss quite dramatically.

In the older child, particularly in the adolescent with untreated plagiocephaly, the bone is not at all malleable. In these types of cases, we will use the same surgical techniques as in the child, where we mark out a new orbital bandeau and also a new forehead using a template. Because of the thickness of the bone, a split-thickness calvarial bone graft will be necessary. After elevating the forehead template, that piece is then split and the inner table is used as patch bone and the outer table used as the forehead piece (see also Chapter 3 for further discussion of the "calvarial split-thickness" technique).

The new orbital bandeau will be also split along the dipolic space, and the outer table will be used as the forehead piece. One can also notch or rib the inner portion of the bone to give it a little more malleability and allow it to fit better into position (Figs. 5–17, 5–18). Once the orbital bandeau is positioned, then the forehead plate can be brought forward and put into position. The excess bone that has been left over will then be used to patch up the defects. In an adolescent or adult skull, it is imperative each of the bony defects be repaired because the bone growth patterns in these older kids is nowhere near as exuberant as in a child. So, every attempt should be made to patch up the holes as best as possible.

An appreciation of each of these various techniques and their use in any of a number of surgical combinations will allow for excellent aesthetic corrections and adequate brain growth. We have found all of these techniques to be most useful in correction of plagiocephaly from infants to adolescents and even adults with traumatic injuries (Figs. 5–19, 5–20).

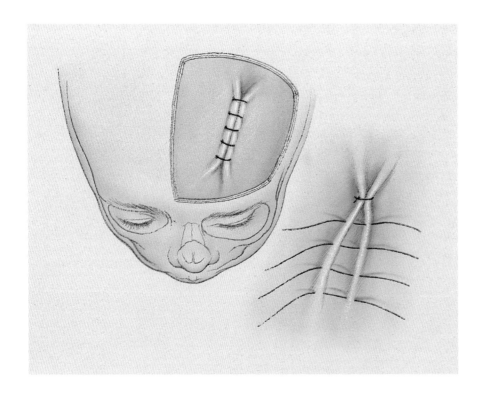

Figure 5–16.   In the case of a plagiocephaly with a prominent frontal boss a useful technique to reduce the prominent boss is dural plication. The technique is illustrated here. By "gripping" the outer dural layer and sewing this in furrow fashion, the prominent boss can be reduced quite dramatically. This provides an easier contour on which to lay the reconstructed forehead.

Figure 5–17. Some useful techniques illustrated here for dealing with an older and thicker skull. Children after the age of 6 months or so lose their bone malleability. Some useful tricks are to place fan cuts in the bone to allow bending around the frontal boss. In this operative slide is also an illustration of the triangular tongue-in-groove used in Figure 5–11. This child had such a prominent slope to the forehead that both a rounding out and triangular tongue-in-groove advancement were needed.

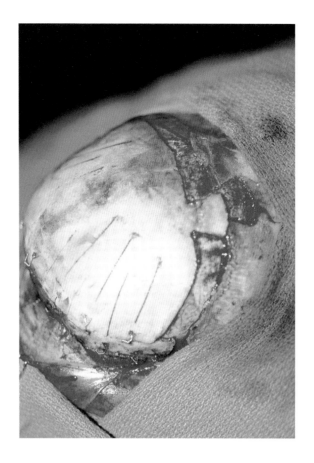

Figure 5–18. An intraoperative view showing the orbital bandeau elevated. Because this was an older child with thicker bone, we have fan notched the inner table to allow more ''bending'' of the bone. This is a useful technique to provide additional malleability to otherwise thick bone.

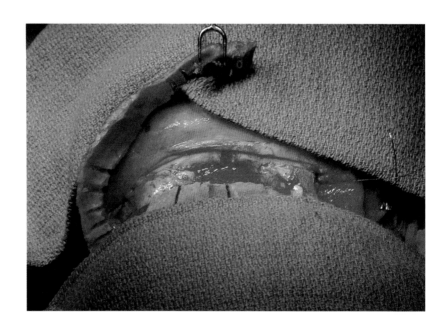

Figure 5-19. A 3-month-old girl with severe right coronal synostosis. The right coronal suture is fused prematurely with a compensatory left frontal boss. There is also deviation of the nasoethmoidal complex, also with asymmetry of the orbital line and orbital dystropia.

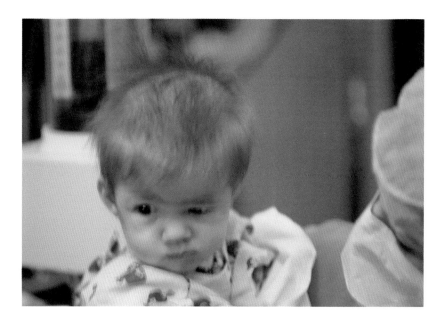

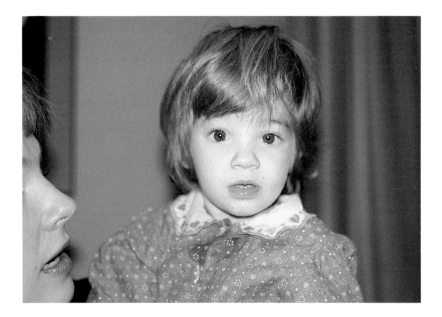

Figure 5-20. The same child as in Figure 5-19 at 1 year postoperative interval showing the cosmetic results obtainable with the techniques described in this chapter.

Scaphocephaly (Sagittal Synostosis)

The treatment of scaphocephaly has been as varied and innovative as the number of surgeons involved in the design of the techniques (Figs. 5–21, 5–22). Scaphocephaly is probably one of the earliest synostoses to be treated on a regular basis, and in particular using the techniques developed by Matson and Ingraham.[10,11] The original technique of Matson is outlined in Figure 5–23. This technique involves a synostectomy either bilateral to the sagittal suture or else taking out the entire sagittal suture. After removing the suture, the edges of the bone are lined with Silastic wrappers to restrict bone growth. The principle behind the use of Silastic was to try and slow down the bone growth. This would then allow a compensatory head growth and reduction of the scaphocephalic look. The problem with this Silastic technique has been that the dura is still quite osteogenic and as a result, despite the Silastic interposition, bone can still reform prematurely. This technique also did not correct the underlying scaphoid shape of the head, so as a result of this failure, a number of techniques have been introduced over the years.

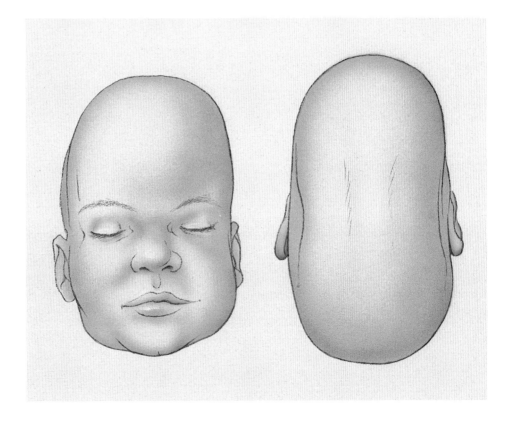

Figure 5–21. A schematic showing the typical features of a scaphocephalic child. The head is elongated in the anteroposterior orientation, leading to a very narrow calvarium. This child also has "waistbanding" of the apex.

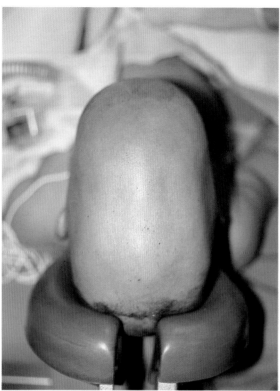

Figure 5–22.   The child in Figure 5–21 here in the operating room, brow up with head resting in a cerebellar headrest. This is our typical operative position, which allows access to both the forehead and calvarium. The head can be flexed even further if more of the occipital region is needed for exposure.

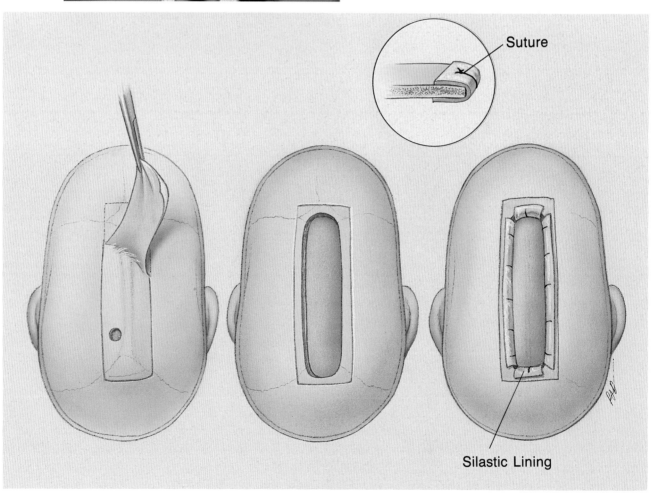

Figure 5–23.   A schematic showing the Silastic technique developed by Matson's group. After the bone is removed, the edges are lined with Silastic.

One of the earliest and most popular techniques was a radical bilateral parietal synostectomy introduced by Luis Schut and his group,[18] shown in Figure 5–24. The technique involves a wide craniosynostectomy incorporating both wide lateral margins and carrying it down close to the base of the skull. This would then allow biparietal-temporal expansion of the brain and skull, giving a more symmetrical comestic result.

A modification of this technique has been introduced by Jane and Pershing,[19] the π-squeeze technique (Figs. 5–25 through 5–29). The principle with this technique is that the surgeon can get a rapid correction of the scaphocephaly with a rounded appearance to the head. The technique is shown in Figures 5–25 through 5–28. The bone cuts are somewhat similar to Schut's technique with the following modifications.[18] A free-floating bone unit over the sagittal suture is kept intact. Advancing this sagittal piece forward up to the forehead bone shortens the longitudinal axis of the head. In cases in which the

Figure 5–24. The Schut technique with wide biparietal bone cuts that then allow the parietal-temporal units to wing out. The cuts have to be carried very low, right to the floor level of the middle fossa.

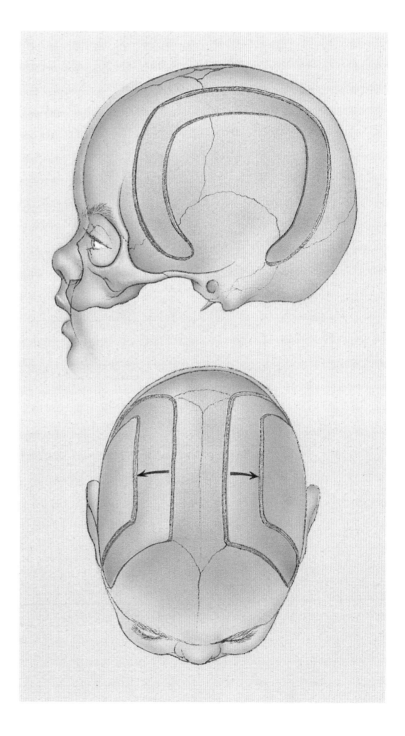

Figure 5–25. The π-squeeze technique illustrated here. After a wide and high bifrontal skin flap is carried forward, the bone cuts are made as illustrated. The sagittal strip is dissected free and moved forward to bring up the back of the skull. If there is a prominent frontal boss, then the frontal unit can be "greensticked" along the orbital rim and moved back. This then moves the lateral plates outward and causes an immediate correction of the scaphocephaly. The insert shows a typical greenstick cut where only the outer table of bone is cut, the inner table is left intact to provide for a hinge.

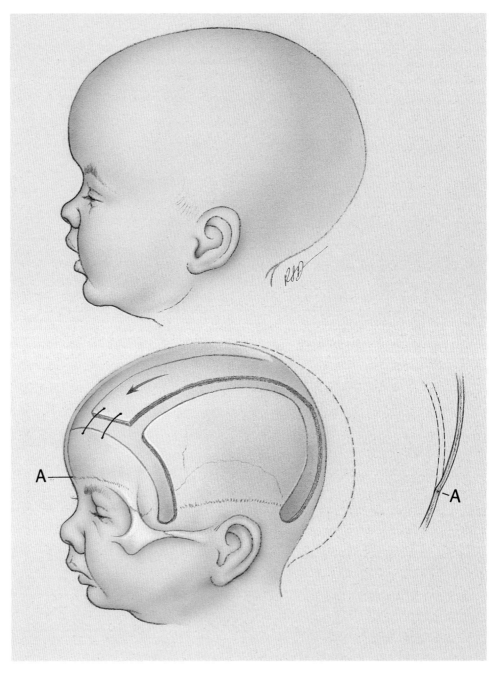

forehead is quite prominent, a greenstick furrow can be placed along the forehead base just superior to the orbital rim. This cut will allow the forehead unit to be "fractured" back and wired to the sagittal unit. By carrying the synostectomies down low and lateral in the temporal region, the biparietal plates can be advanced laterally (Figs. 5–27, 5–28). The end result of all of this is an excellent cosmetic reshaping of the head (Fig. 5–29). Both of these techniques can lead to extensive bleeding from the bone. Therefore the surgical team has to be prepared for blood transfusions. Meticulous technique will keep the bleeding minimal.

Another technique that has been popularized by the French is the "transposition technique"[13] (Fig. 5–30). In the case of a child with severe scaphocephaly with a "waistbanding" of the head, the transposition technique has been useful for remodeling the head. As shown in Figure 5–30, a marking out of various bone plates is done. These units are elevated and then repositioned. In the top figure is the head as it would appear with severe scaphocephaly. The various segments are marked out; these segments can then be removed as a unit piece. Usually, the

Figure 5–26. An intraoperative photograph showing the forehead after the π cuts have been made. The greenstick cut is evident at the base of the forehead.

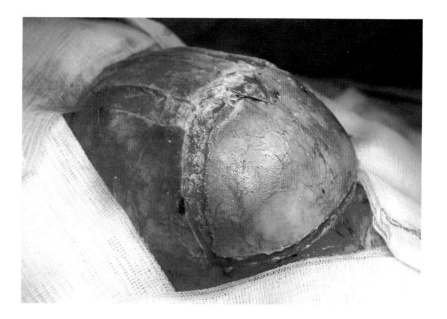

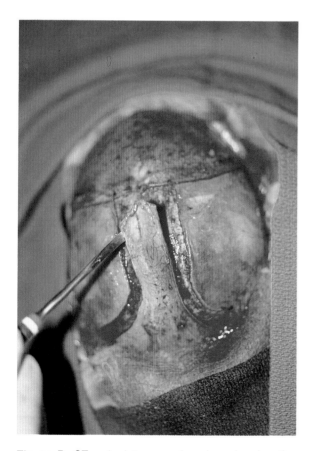

Figure 5–27. An intraoperative view showing the sagittal strip being elevated off the sagittal sinus just prior to forward advancement.

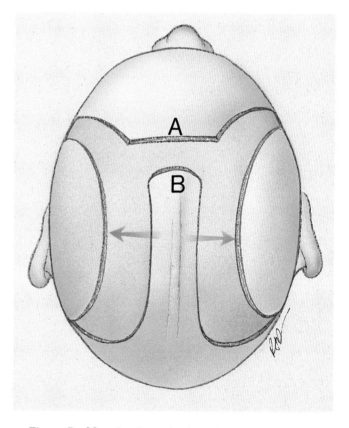

Figure 5–28. A schematic view of Figure 5–27 showing the various bone cuts that are made in the π-squeeze technique. After dissection, the point labeled "B" is advanced to point "A" and then wired into position (this is also shown in Figure 5–25). The parietotemporal plates then move laterally, as shown by the arrow direction. This movement causes a correction in the longitudinal axis to give a more rounded appearance.

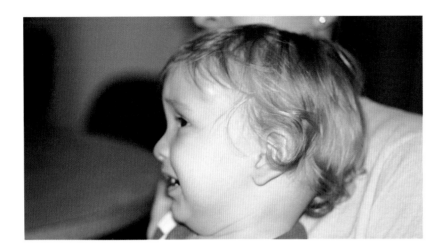

Figure 5-29. Postoperative appearance of the patient in Figure 5-22 at 10 months. In this patient the π-squeeze technique was used as illustrated in Figures 5-26 and 5-27.

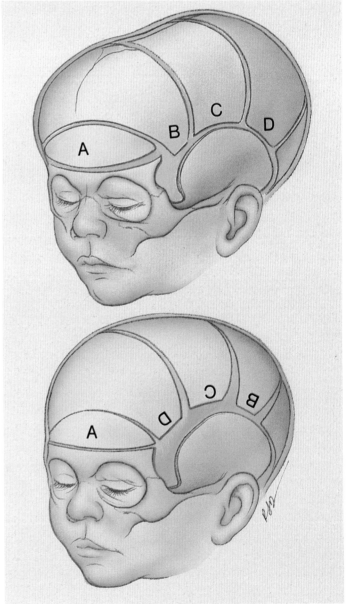

A

B

Figure 5-30. **A, B:** The transposition technique illustrated here showing the pieces labeled along with where the osteotomies are made. **B:** The patient after the transpositions have been completed. The piece labeled ''C'' in **B** has actually been turned around. There are any number of variations that can be used here. It is again up to the surgeon to try out various positions to see which is most aesthetically pleasing.

portion of bone over the frontal and occipital regions tends to have the most reasonable shape. By reversing these units, the surgeon can correct the prominent frontal bossing that occurs. Sometimes if the "waistband" piece, marked C in this diagram, is reversed, it will compensate for the constriction that has occurred. This is only one of a number of examples of various types of transposition techniques that can be used. It is really up to the ingenuity of the surgeon to decide where the pieces will fit best. The technique requires moving around the various units until the best contour is achieved.

Another technique that has been advanced but that has not been as popular with surgeons is the "morcellation technique." In this case, the surgeon removes the entire calvarium, as small pieces of bone. These pieces are relaid into position. The problem with this technique is that you get little control over the contour, plus you leave a very fragile head during the growing period. For these reasons, we have not been strong advocates of this particular technique.

Trigonocephaly (Metopic Synostosis)

The treatment of trigonocephaly incorporates many of the techniques that have been discussed in earlier sections. However, because of the combination of eye abnormalities (hypotelorism), our group has been incorporating both the orbital/lateral advancement and the metopic forehead correction in a single stage. We will review some of those techniques in this section.

The trigonocephalic child, as shown in Figures 5–31, 5–32, has the typical keel shape or pointed brow. This case is due to premature fusion of the metopic suture. In addition, it has been our experience that the coronal sutures are also fused simultaneously in a very high incidence of these children. As a result, one sees a child with a keel-shaped head with a "pinched" forehead look (Fig. 5–31). Thus, these children can be hypotelorotic with the eyes being too close together. We have devised a combined lateral orbital advancement along with a new orbital bandeau and forehead reconstruction. In

Figures 5–32, 5–33, 5–36 we have outlined the two important parts of this procedure. After the routine bifrontal skin flap is rotated forward, we then mark out the orbital bandeau over the top of calvarium; this piece is going to replace the now markedly narrow forehead piece (Figs. 5–32, 5–33, 5–34). The original orbital bandeau cannot be used because of the hypoteleorism of the eyes plus the firm metopic suture that is still present. The old bandeau is actually discarded or used later as strut pieces. In Figure 5–32A is shown a typical child with the trigonocephaly, and in B is the marked area of donor bone units. Using a forehead template, a new forehead piece is drawn out (Fig. 5–33). In Figures 5–34, 5–35 the forehead orbital bandeau and forehead piece have been removed and wired together to provide the typical contour that is needed (Fig. 5–35).

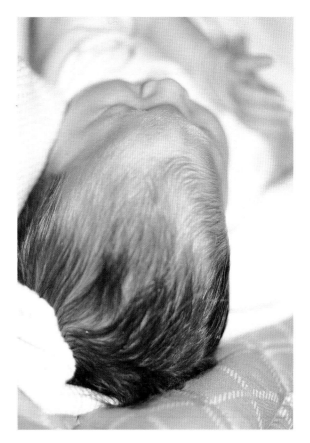

Figure 5–31. A typical case of a metopic premature fusion with resultant "keel-shaped" forehead. In addition, hypotelorism developed in this child.

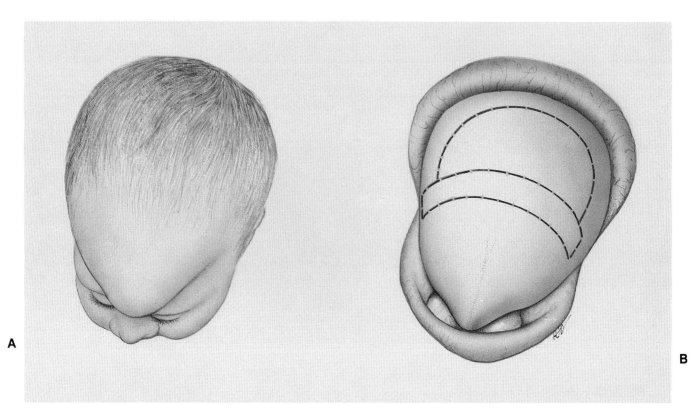

A   B

Figure 5–32.   **A, B:** Schematic of the child in Figure 5–31 showing the outline of the bone cuts for harvesting a new orbital bandeau and forehead. A wide bifrontal skin flap has to be moved to provide adequate exposure of the operative field.

Figure 5–33.   An intraoperative view of the head with the bone cuts marked out in methylene blue. This compares with the schematic in Figure 5–32B.

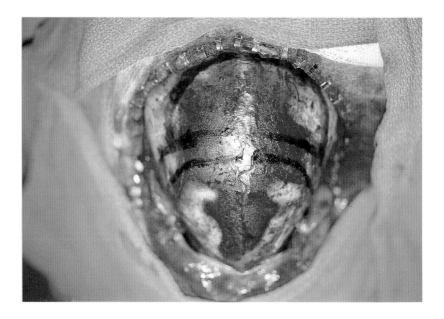

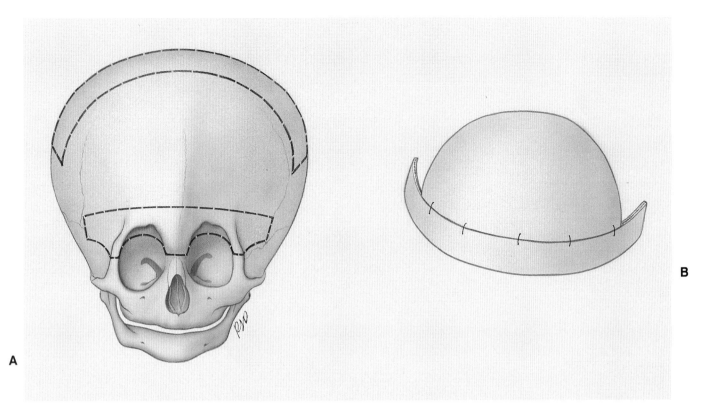

A

B

Figure 5–34. Since the orbital bandeau is foreshortened in metopic cases, this unit is not reusable. This bandeau is taken out in the standard fashion and either discarded or used as strut pieces **(A). B:** The reconstruction of the newly harvested orbital bandeau and forehead unit.

Figure 5–35. The orbital bandeau and forehead unit have been wired together just prior to replacing.

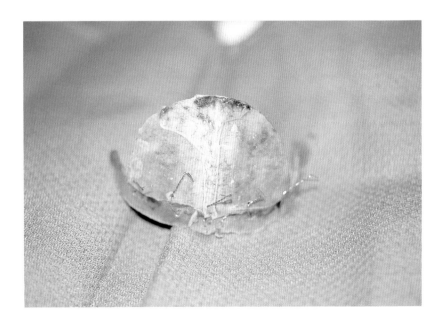

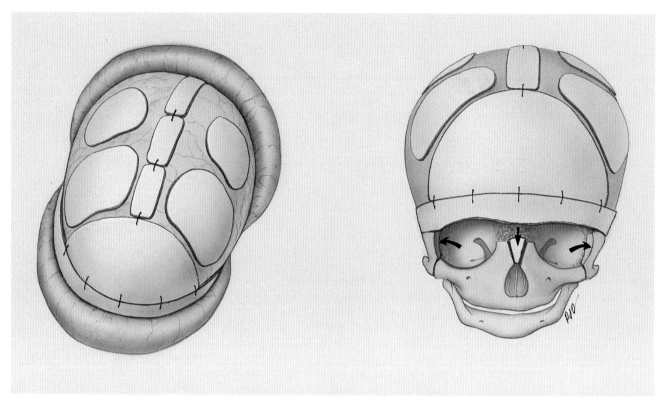

Figure 5–36.   A schematic showing the reconstruction, including the nasal split and lateral orbital advancement. The wedge of bone in the nasal septum is in place. In addition, the calvarium has been reconstructed in a mosaic fashion using the remaining bone. The sagittal piece is very important for both protection of the sagittal sinus and preventing "towering" of the calvarium.

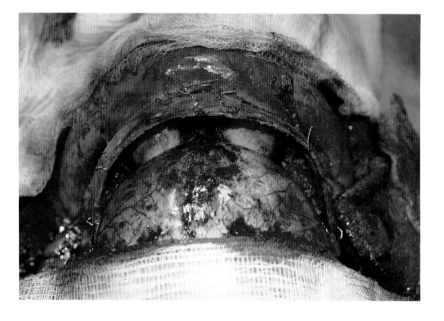

Figure 5–37.   An operative view looking down on the forehead and repositioning of the orbital bandeau. The top of both orbits are visible plus the advancement space between the dura and orbital bandeau stands out. The interorbital distance has been increased by 13 mm in this case.

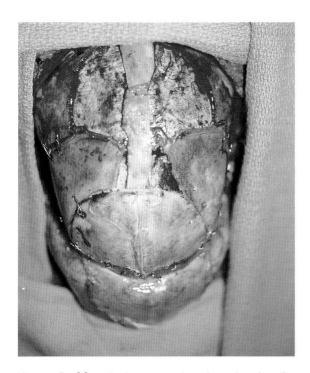

Figure 5–38. An intraoperative view showing the equivalent picture of Figure 5–36 (left side) with the bone units in final position. The new forehead and orbital advancement have given a satisfactory reconstruction of this metopic asymmetry.

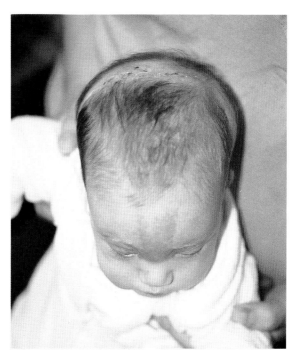

Figure 5–39. The patient in Figure 5–31 at 1 month postoperative, showing a normal interpupillary distance and correction of the forehead keel.

The surgeon can also elect to correct the hypotelorism at the same time; Figure 5–36B shows the technique that we used. The bifrontal forehead skin flap has to be carried way forward down to the nose, exposing well below the nasal suture line. In addition, both zygomas need to be exposed to well below the zygoma suture. The midnasal bone is fractured and separated out in a lateral direction. A bone wedge is inserted to keep this unit laterally separated (illustrated in Figure 5–36B). The lateral orbital walls are advanced laterally by fracturing through the zygomatic arch. The superior orbital roof cut is presented from the previous craniotomy when removing the orbital bandeau. This lateral orbital unit is then fractured outward (Fig. 5–36B). The combination of these two techniques allows an increase in the interpupillary distance by at least 1 to 1.5 cm (Fig. 5–37). The calvarium is then replaced together in a series of interposition bone grafts, as shown in Figures 5–36A, 5–38. Using what bone is left, the most important piece is the one that goes up over the sagittal sinus. The calvarium should also be covered with bone, leaving the lateral convexity open if there is a shortage of bone; this prevents the towering (turricephaly) that can occur (Fig. 5–39).

The older technique of just removing the metopic suture did not correct the hypotelorism. In addition, this technique did not deal with the often commonly associated fused coronal sutures, and for this reason the single synostectomy technique is not reasonable in this syndrome. This combined forehead and lateral orbital advancement allows a single-stage reconstruction, which provides excellent aethestic results.

Lambdoidal Synostosis

This section will deal with the treatment of unilateral and bilateral synostosis of the lambdoidal sutures. When lambdoidal synostosis occurs, a child develops a very typical-looking appearance (Fig. 5–40). In the simpler unilateral lambdoidal synostosis, one gets a flattening of one side of the head, which in most cases can easily be ignored because it does not lead to growth constriction. Since the asymmetry is in the back of the head, this usually does not lead to major cosmetic problems, particularly when the child develops a full head of hair. There are situations when the synostosis can be significant enough that torticollis and malalignment of the ears occur due to premature fusion through the skull base. In severe cases there can be severe rotational deformation of the petrous ridges. In these more serious situations it is appropriate to consider a craniofacial reconstruction for correction.

A useful surgical approach in unilateral lambdoidal synostosis is called the "fan technique" (Figs. 5–41, 5–42). A biparietal skin flap is rotated with the child in the prone position. A craniectomy is marked out that encompasses the entire area of flattening and the margins are continued out even more generously from that. One must remember that this is an area frought with complications because of the torcular Herophili, sagittal and lateral sinuses. The surgeon has to be extremely careful in elevating the bone flap so as not to injure the sinuses. In young children, the amount of fibrosis between the bone sutures and the underlying dura is not that great; therefore elevation of the bone flap can be done in a straightforward fashion. After elevation of the bone flap (see Fig. 5–42), a number of fan cuts are placed in a radial fashion around the bone flap. After the fan cuts, the bone is molded in the position wanted to form a more appropriate contour. Once accomplished, the fan cuts are then wired together giving the conformity desired (see Fig. 5–43). The bone flap is then wired back into position. This is an easy and very straightforward technique for dealing with unilateral lambdoidal synostosis (Fig. 5–44).

Children with bilateral lambdoidal synostosis are a more complicated problem and these children can end up with a number of craniofacial deformities (Fig. 5–45). It has been our experience that children with lambdoidal synostosis, if not treated early, can have severe ear anomalies, particularly with petrous ridge anomalies, so that one ear can end up lower than the other. Plus the ear can be displaced forward or backward in relation to the opposite ear. For these reasons, it is important to be very aggressive in treating these deformities early on. The typical suture synostectomy is not a useful technique in this type of problem because it does not correct the underlying abnormality, particularly the widened biparietal distance.

A commonly used surgical technique is a modification of the transposition technique developed by the French.[13] As shown in Figure 5–46, after a biparietal skin flap, two bone units la-

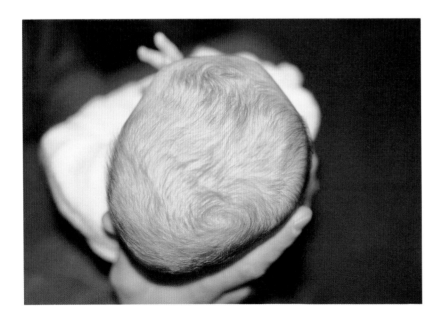

Figure 5–40. Typical example of a child with unilateral lambdoidal synostosis affecting the right side. As a result of this premature fusion, the child's right ear was displaced forward and upward. The compensatory bossing on the left side increased the asymmetry and this was carried through the skull base and both petrous ridges.

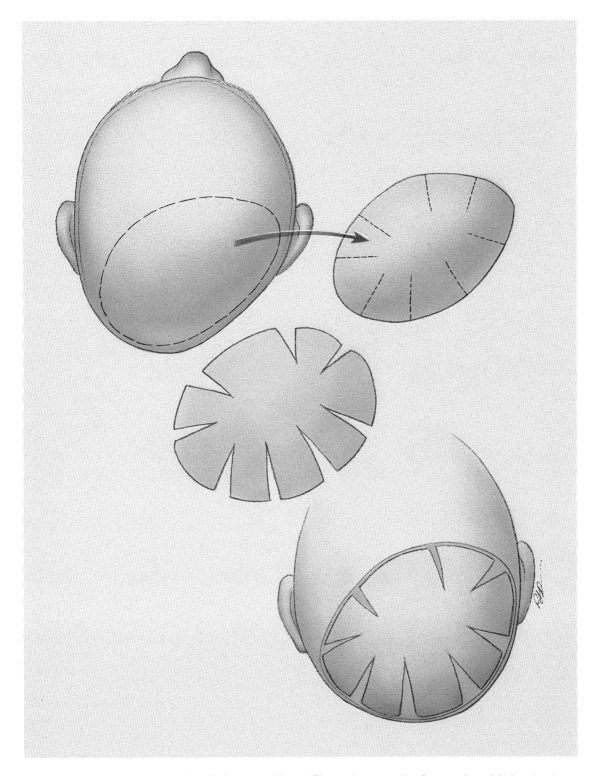

Figure 5–41. "Fan technique" diagramed here. The region over the flattened occipital region is marked out. This unit of bone is then elevated out and taken off the field. The radial fan cuts are placed around the borders, as diagramed here.

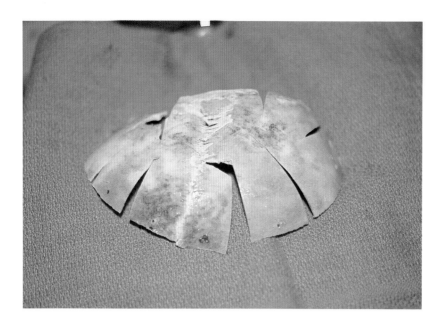

Figure 5–42. The occipital bone after the fan cuts have been completed.

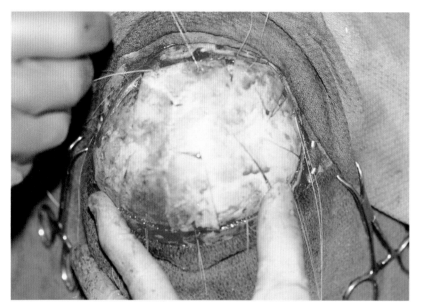

Figure 5–43. The fanned bone is then molded into the contour desired and wired into position. The pericranium is laid down over the cuts and the skin flap replaced.

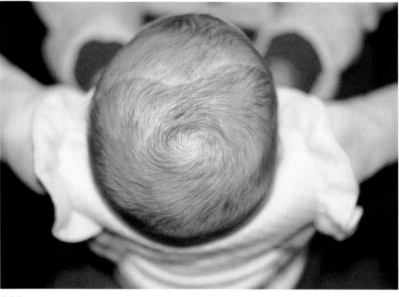

Figure 5–44. The child in Figure 5–40 after surgery at 6 weeks postoperative.

Figure 5–45. A child with severe bilateral lambdoidal synostosis with constriction of growth in the anteroposterior axis. The lambdoidal sutures were actually inverted in this child. On facial view, the patient had a significantly widened biparietal distance to allow for compensatory brain growth.

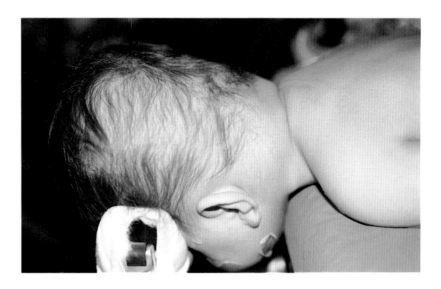

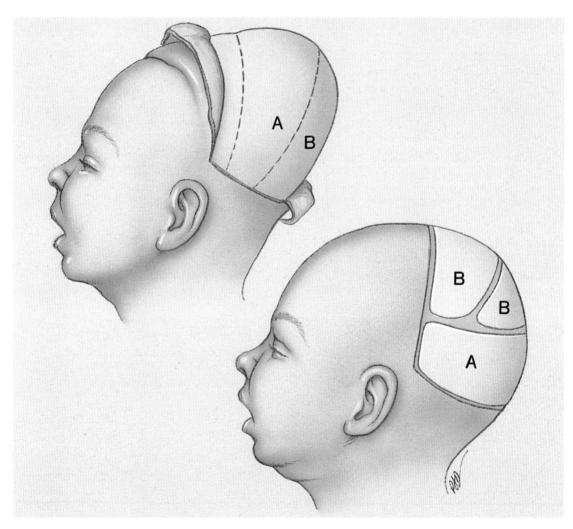

Figure 5–46. A schematic view of the "transposition technique." The principle here is to remove the occipital and parietal bones in such a fashion as to allow reconstruction with more normally contoured bone. The unit labeled "A" will form the new occipital unit. The piece labeled "B" can be transposed to "A" position or even broken up into smaller units to make a mosaic reconstruction. All of these options are available and up to the discretion of the surgeon.

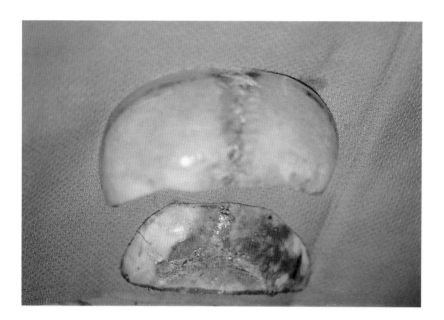

Figure 5–47. The two units of bone labeled "A" and "B" in Figure 5–46 are here removed and placed off the field to be transposed into the desired contour.

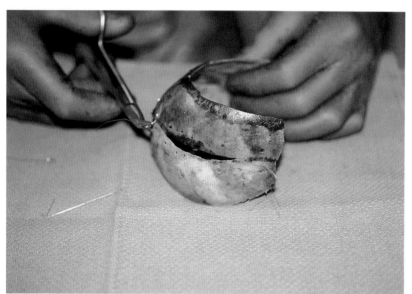

Figure 5–48. The surgeon wiring into position the transposed units of bone. In this case the transposition was successful with just two units. In many cases the second piece will have to be cut up and then reconstructed in a mosaic fashion to get a better contour.

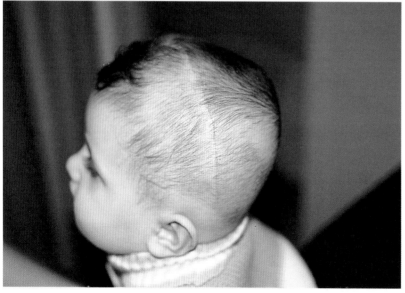

Figure 5–49. The patient in Figure 5–45 at 3 weeks postoperative after a transposition technique.

beled A and B are marked out. Bone piece A, which now is over the biparietal area, will be the unit transposed and placed over the occipital region to form the new posterior border of the head. Elevation of these flaps has to be done carefully because of the sinuses that underlie them. However, with the use of the high-speed drill system, it is relatively easy to elevate the flaps (Figs. 5–47, 5–48). A useful trick is to elevate both sides together and meet at the sagittal suture line. The flaps can be bent easily ("gull-winged") at that point and elevated off of the sagittal sinus without much difficulty. The same applies particularly to the occipital bone, which can be elevated as far down as the foramen magnum, if necessary. Take these two units and reposition them, as in Figures 5–46 and 5–48. The bone units are tongue-in-grooved to the temporal squamous bone and wired into position. After the contours have been selected that are appropriate, the pericranium and skin flaps are then replaced.

Postoperatively, the child has to be kept either on the stomach or rotated from side to side. Our biggest problem has been with children who flip on their back and put undue pressure on these bone flaps after they have been repositioned. On occasion, we have made helmets, contoured and molded to be placed into position to help in the correction. The important surgical consideration with this surgical technique is that both lambdoidal sutures and the sagittal suture have to be incorporated in the transposition because this is where the severe constriction will occur, and these have to be corrected (Fig. 5–49).

Pansynostosis (Multiple Suture Closure)

In the treatment of craniofacial disorders, the one problem that has been among the most complicated is that of children born with multiple suture fusion, "pansynostosis or cloverleaf skulls." The other term commonly used is kleeblattschädel. These children can be medical emergencies because of the severe bone vault constriction. This constriction causes growth delay that results in significant developmental delay to the children. These children need to be

evaluated early, and surgery is commonly done within the first 2 months of life.

The techniques used in the treatment of cloverleaf skulls have been as varied as simple suture synostectomies to full calvarial morcellations. A group in France led by Maurice Choux has advocated the complete removal of the calvarium itself, leaving no bone behind. Choux has found that with intact periosteum and dura, the children will form new calvarial bone.

In multiple suture fusions, a useful technique is a transposition-type technique with complete removal of the calvarium and then restructuring of it along the normal contour lines. In Figure 5–50 is an example of a child with severe pansynostosis with multiple suture fusions. On skull x-ray, this child had severe thumbprinting from underlying increased intracranial pres-

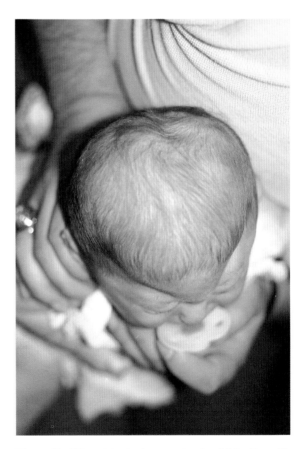

Figure 5–50. A typical example of a child with multiple sutures closed prematurely. Besides the cloverleaf shape, it can be appreciated the number of "lumps and bumps" that can occur over the calvarium. There are places where the bone is usually quite thinned and the brain is attempting to break through in an effort to decompress.

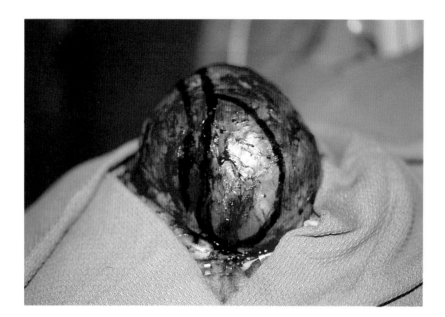

Figure 5–51. Intraoperative view of the calvarium after the bifrontal skin flap is rotated. This is a lateral view of the calvarium and the methylene blue markings are where the new orbital bandeau and forehead unit are going to be harvested. This position of the forehead unit turned out to be the only normally shaped piece of bone in the calvarium.

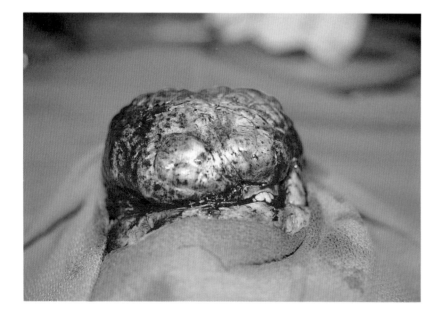

Figure 5–52. After complete removal of the calvarium, it is easy to appreciate the severe deformity that occurs with brain as it attempts to expand in the normal growth pattern. The surface of this brain was a number of valleys and grooves where the brain had attempted to break out through thinned bone. In a number of spots the bone was actually absent due to erosion from increased intracranial pressure.

Figure 5–53.   The various units of bone that have been harvested are then wired into position. In this case the orbital bandeau and forehead were constructed first and the remaining bone was used to complete the calvarium. In cases of severe pansynostosis it is always interesting how little bone is available for reconstruction secondary to the growth erosion.

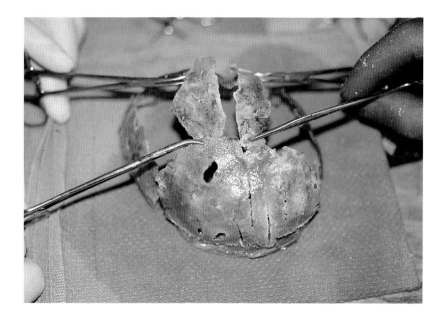

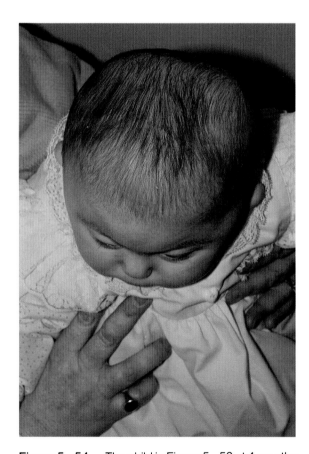

Figure 5–54.   The child in Figure 5–50 at 4 months postoperatively. Repeat skull x-rays at 6 months showed no bone mottling and almost complete calvarial regrowth of bone.

sure. We estimated that over 50% of her skull bone was lost due to bone erosion secondary to pressure. At surgery, the child was placed in the prone position with the head hyperextended. The entire calvarium was removed from the ears up. These tend to be difficult procedures to do, because as a result of the bone mottling, the bone tends to be extremely uneven. Technically, it is hard to move a craniotome along the uneven bony surfaces (see Figs. 5–51, 5–52). In these types of situations, we have found a high-speed drill system with small footplates like the Midas Rex to be particularly valuable. With great care the entire calvarium can be removed without injury to the sinuses. Once that is done, the bone units are taken off of the table and put back together in the position that most approximates the normal calvarium (Fig. 5–53). Because of the increased intracranial pressure and significant bone erosion in this child, large defects of bone are left behind, but these will fill in with time. At the completion, the bifrontal skin flap was closed in a routine fashion, taking great care to lay out completely the pericranium. For these children, we make molded helmets as additional protection. Helmets also act additionally as molding forces for the calvarium. Interestingly, the postoperative skull films in pansynostosis will show complete resolution of the thumb-printing over a period of about 6 months if there is adequate room for brain growth (Fig. 5–54).

Conclusion

The purpose of this chapter has been to show some of the various techniques available for treatment of the more complicated craniofacial disorders. Although this chapter has been broken up into various sections, each of these techniques can be interchangeably used with the various syndromes. When incorporated with children with Crouzon's and Apert's Syndrome, as discussed by Dr. Argamaso (Chapter 6), it is now easily appreciated that one can take the entire calvarium and midface apart. Then, depending on the aesthetics and necessary growth dynamics, the various units can be symmetrically replaced. The techniques that are being used are quite safe and when done by an experienced craniofacial team can provide excellent cosmetic results.

References

1. Hundt M. Antrologium de hominis dignitate. Leipzig, 1501.
2. Dryander J. Anatomie Capitis Humani. Marburg: 1537.
3. Vesalius A. De humani corporis fabrica. Basel: Oporinis, 1543.
4. Croce GAD. Cirugia Universale e Perfetta. Venetia: Giordana Ziletti, 1583.
5. Lannelungue, OM. De la craniotome dans la microcephalie. CR Acad Sci 1890;110:1382–6.
6. Lannelungue OM. Craniectome dans les Microcephale. In: Congrés der Chirurgiens francais, 1891.
7. Dennis FS. System of Surgery. Philadelphia: Lea, 1895. See volume 2, pages 715–721.
8. Lane LC. Surgery of the Head and Neck. San Francisco: privately printed, 1896.
9. MacEwen W. The Growth of Bone. Observations on Osteogenesis. Glasgow: MacLehose, 1912:142–5.
10. Ingraham FD, Alexander E, Matson DD. Clinical studies in craniosynostosis: Analysis of fifty cases and description of a method of surgical treatment. Surgery 1948;24:518–41.
11. Matson DD. Neurosurgery of infancy and childhood. 2nd ed. Springfield, IL: Charles C Thomas, 1969.
12. Mount LA. Premature closure of sutures of cranial vault—a plea for early recognition and early operation. NY State J Med 1947;47:270–276.
13. Marchac D, Renier D. Craniofacial Surgery for Craniosynostosis. Boston: Little, Brown, 1982.
14. Epstein F, McCarthy JG, Coccaro PJ. Prophylactic craniofacial surgery. Child's Brain 1979;5:204–15.
15. Marchac D. Craniofacial Surgery. Proceedings of the First International Congress of the International Society of Cranio-Maxillo-Facial Surgery. Berlin: Springer-Verlag, 1987.
16. Tessier P. Craniofacial surgery in syndromic craniosynostosis. In: Cohen MM Jr (ed): Craniosynostosis Diagnosis, Evaluation, and Management. New York: Raven Press, 1986:321–411.
17. Tessier P. The definitive plastic surgical treatment of the severe facial deformities of craniofacial dysostosis. Crouzon's and Apert's diseases. Plast Reconstr Surg 1971;48:419–42.
18. Stein SC, Schut L. Management of scaphocephaly. Surg Neurol 1977;7:153–5.
19. Jane JA, Pershing JA. Neurosurgical treatment of craniosynostosis. In: Cohen MM Jr (ed): Craniosynostosis Diagnosis, Evaluation, and Management. New York: Raven Press, 1986:249–320.

SIX

RAVELO V. ARGAMASO, M.D.

Congenital Facial Disorders: Surgical Techniques

This chapter will deal with some of the recent developments in plastic and craniofacial surgery. Techniques for surgery about the orbit and midface have became especially important as neurosurgeons have become more aggressive in their management of skull base and anterior fossa tumors. These surgical techniques now often play an important role in facial remodeling after severe facial injuries that commonly occur in motor vehicle accidents. As craniofacial teams involving plastic surgery and neurosurgery become more prevalent, these techniques will become essential in the modern management of the more complex skull base tumors. In addition, more complex surgical techniques are available to deal with injury of the craniofacial complex along with the more common congenital craniofacial disorders.

Craniofacial deformities are prevalent among neonates with multiple birth defects. They are now seen in increasing numbers in craniofacial centers whose scope of interest includes congenital facial disorders with clefting, midface deformities, and orbital abnormalities. During the past two decades, Tessier's innovative and elaborate craniofacial reconstructions have attracted universal attention.[1,2] These resulted in a re-markable physical transformation and a significant psychologic improvement in the patient's self-perception.

For purposes of describing the surgical strategies performed successfully in correcting some of the more common deformities affecting specific areas of the face and cranium, an arbitrary regionalization of the craniofacial territory will be outlined. It should be emphasized, however, that because a deforming process occurring at one region can influence the development of neighboring structures and eventually can even alter the configuration of the rest of the craniofacial skeleton, a combination of these surgical maneuvers may be called for. Hence, in dealing with a more complex craniofacial malformation, a modification in the operations may be developed, depending on the ingenuity of the surgical team.

Cranium and Forehead

Cranioplasty for calvarial and forehead deformities is discussed in Chapter 3. It will be described only insofar as it relates to correction of the orbits.

109

Orbits and Interorbital Area

Hypoplasia of the orbits may be caused by a primary deficiency in the bony constituents or by a congenital absence or underdevelopment of the globes. Premature fusion of the frontal sutures of the cranium are associated with orbital displacements. These altered relationships can remain stationary at best, or they can worsen with growth.

Exorbitism

Protruding eyes, a sequela of craniofacial dysostosis, occur because of a shallowness of the sockets. They are not secondary to an enlargement of the socket contents, which is a distinguishing feature of hyperthyroidism. In extreme cases, the eyes are prolapsed, necessitating an immediate tarsorrhaphy in order to protect the corneas for vision.

Corrective surgery for exorbitism per se consists of an anterior expansion of the orbit. When proptosis is a consequence of craniofacial dysostosis, the forehead and midface are moved forward with the rims of the orbits. The osteotomies may be undertaken at two different levels, i.e., fronto-orbital and midfacial, and executed in two stages. In the first stage, the advancement of the frontal bone with the upper half of the orbits is performed early in infancy (3 to 6 months). It is followed by the next stage, the advancement of the midface with the lower half of the orbits, after age 4 years or preferably during adolescence. Others advocate combining these two procedures at the same operative session[3] or by performing a single fronto-orbital-facial (monobloc) advancement.[4] The greatest obstacle to an outright endorsement of this more audacious procedure is the risk of an intracranial sepsis via the potentially open communication between the nasal and anterior cranial compartments.

As described in Chapter 5, fronto-orbital advancement is recommended to be done early to relieve intracranial hypertension, to improve the contour of the frontal cranium, and to diminish the prominence of the eyes. Midfacial advancement complements the aesthetic effects of fronto-orbital surgery: to alleviate exorbitism and to bring the maxilla into a more favorable balance with the mandible. Restoration of the maxillary and mandibular relationships enhances masticatory and dentolabial speech functions. The operation will be elaborated on later in the chapter.

Rarely, exorbitism will manifest itself without a discernable midfacial deformity. Dental occlusion is usually normal (Fig. 6-1).

In such a condition, correction is accomplished by an orbitonasal osteotomy through bicoronal, lower lid, and buccal incisions. Through these openings, the orbits and midface are subperiosteally divested of their overlying soft tissues. The outline of the osteotomy initiated across the radix nasi extends to the medial orbital walls above the level of the lachrimal fossa, skirts it, and turns inferiorly toward and across the floor. At about the frontozygomatic junction, the lateral orbital rim is cut in a step fashion. The spur that develops in the inferior segment abuts against the rim of the superior segment after the lower part of the orbit is advanced. The osteotomy of the lateral wall is joined with the osteotomy of the floor. Outside the orbits, the lateral cut continues on the body of the zygoma and then proceeds medially toward the pyriform aperture of the nose. The process is repeated on the opposite side. Finally, the nasal septum is cut after a submucus dissection. Having connected all the osteotomy lines, the deep bony connections of thin bones are easily fractured as the orbitonasal unit is mobilized in a forward and slightly downward direction. Autogenous bone blocks obtained from the ilium are impacted into the nasofrontal and zygomatic defects and secured with interosseous wires. Split rib grafts are also laid over the gaps created over the maxillae and orbital floors. A successful "take" of these grafts will maintain the orbitonasal advancement and prevent relapse. Additional strips of rib grafts are placed and wired to the supraorbital rims. Thus, the anterior expansion of the orbit corrects the disparity between the globe size and the sockets that contain them.

It should be emphasized that the safety of the globes, lachrimal system, and the neuromuscular bundles are paramount during any orbital dissection. Hence, the periorbita are kept intact and a safe distance from the optic foramena,

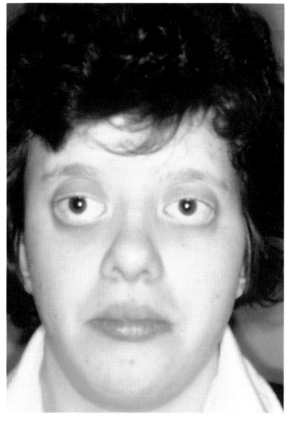

A

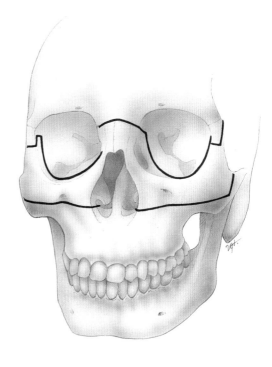

Exorbitism   B

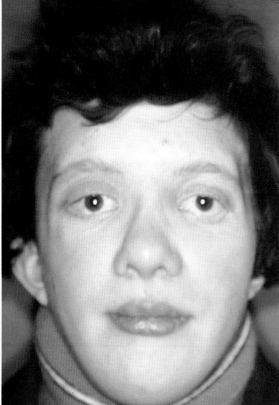

C

Figure 6–1.   **A:** Preoperative appearance showing pronounced exorbitism but with normal dental occlusion. **B:** Outline of the orbitonasal osteotomy to allow for correction of exorbitism. **C:** Postoperative result at 7 months after orbitonasal advancement.

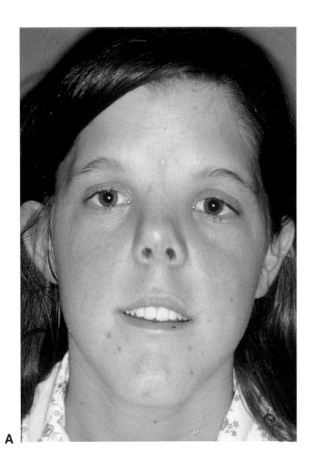

A

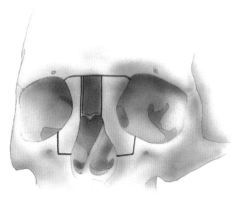

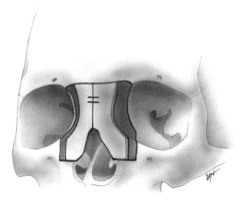

B

Figure 6–2. **A:** An adolescent female with mild hypertelorism. **B:** Outline of the osteotomies performed of the medial orbital walls. This technique also involves a removal of a central segment from the nasal dorsum. *(Figure Continues.)*

which are guarded at all times. Although morbidity with intraorbital surgery is low, some procedures have led to serious consequences.[5,6]

An osteotomy that inadvertently extends to the cribriform plate invariably intrudes into the anterior cranial fossa. The possibility of a dural tear should be ruled out and appropriate treatment instituted. This operation is not advocated for a young patient whose tooth buds are ensconced very high up in the maxilla.

Hyperteleorbitism

In common usage, hypertelorism means the condition in which the eyes are widely separated. Hyperteleorbitism seems a more proper

Figure 6–2 *(continued).*   **C:** Postoperative result at a 3-year follow-up.

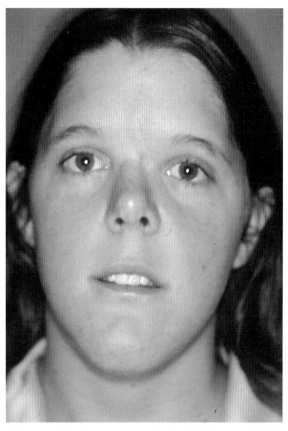

C

designation for a true lateral displacement of the orbits, resulting in an exaggerated distance between the eyes. Almost always, this condition is characterized by a widening of the nasal bridge. Normal measurements between the anterior lachrymal crests in Caucasian adults range from 18.5 to 29.9 mm for females and from 19.5 to 30.7 mm for males. Greater measurements result in a noticeable separation classified as mild (30 to 34 mm), moderate (34 to 40 mm), and severe (over 40 mm). Severity increases with the divergence of the orbital axis, although the distance between their apices (optic foramena) may remain normal. A marked orbital separation impairs eye movements, which brings about the loss of binocularity and convergence. Congenital hyperteleorbitism is not an independent entity, but is associated with a median or paramedian cleft with or without a meningocele. (Examples of hyperteleorbitism in nasoencephalocoeles are shown in Chapter 4). It may accompany some forms of craniofacial dysostosis. The ethmoid labryinth expands and the cribriform plate descends to a lower plane.

Masking procedures on soft tissues may be elected instead of orbital surgery for the mild forms. These rely on creating an illusion of the eyes being closer, by obliterating the epicanthal folds, by drawing the eyebrows medially nearer to each other, and by narrowing the nasal pyramid.[7] Ideally, the best results are achieved by the removal of a central block of nasal bridge with the anterior ethmoids and moving the orbits medially. The cribriform plate may be sacrificed or preserved.[8-11] In the milder forms of hyperteleorbitism, a less extensive operation consists of translocation of only the medial walls in conjunction with narrowing of the nasal bridge.

Since the dorsal midline forms the peak of the nasal elevation, removal of the central section lowers the nasal pyramid. A bone graft is therefore needed to restore the height of the reconstructed nose. Paramedian resections of the nasal bones offer an alternative for narrowing the nose, without changing its profile.[12]

Despite the advantage of a hidden scar from a bicoronal incision, some patients are appalled by its length and will opt for a shorter incision over the glabella and nose. One such patient was a 17-year-old female. At age 5 years, she underwent a corrective rhinoplasty that failed to correct a mild hyperteleorbitism (Fig. 6–2).

The nasal bones, glabella, and orbital walls were dissected subperiosteally through the lower lid and nasoglabellar skin incisions. Exposure of the anterior surface of the maxilla and pyriform apertures was performed through an upper buccal sulcus incision. The osteotomy was started across the root of the nose (Fig. 6–2A). A central section of the nasal bone, 6 mm wide and corresponding to the degree of narrowing desired, was removed. The osteotomy was continued on the medial orbital wall above the lachrimal fossa, past the line of the equator of the globe, and then turned inferiorly toward the floor. The inferior orbital rim was then cut medial to the inferior orbital fissure and infraorbital foramen, traversing the nasal process of the maxilla onward, to the base of the pyriform aperture. This procedure was repeated on the other side. The bony septum was partially resected and the anterior ethmoids exenterated. The medial orbital walls in continuity with their nasal bones were then displaced to the midline and wired to each other and to the glabella. The nasal dorsum was rebuilt with a rib graft anchored to the glabella. Medial canthopexies were performed. A septal cartilage was fashioned to support the columella and project the tip. Bone blocks were burred to conform to the inner surfaces of the lateral walls of the orbits and to keep the globes displaced permanently in their new positions. Finally, a Z-plasty was performed to lengthen the skin on the dorsum of the nose (Fig. 6–2C). Alternatively, these osteotomies, when extended to include the lateral orbital walls, encompass a U-shaped segment of the orbits, which brings the globes along with them when they are shifted medially.

The more severe expression of hyperteleorbitism is corrected successfully only in conjunction with a frontal craniotomy. The collaboration of the neurosurgeon and the plastic surgeon has made the surgical correction of this seemingly formidable deformity possible, with an extremely good prognosis and a reasonable degree of safety.

A 12-year-old girl with a frontonasal dysplasia and a marked hyperteleorbitism is shown in Figure 6–3A. Her interorbital distance between anterior lachrimal crests was 45 mm. A frontal scalp flap was developed and was split in the midline in anticipation of a skin reduction. A bone flap was removed 2.5 cm above the superior orbital rims. The dura was freed and the brain retracted to visualize the anterior cranial fossa. Filaments from the olfactory bulb were cut and the dural openings closed with sutures. Subperiosteal elevation of the scalp flaps was continued over the orbital rims into the orbits to a distance just past the equators of the globes (Fig. 6–3B).

A horizontal osteotomy made 1.5 cm above the superior orbital rims left a narrow band of forehead bone attached to the cranium. Below this bandeau, a 3.5 cm wide central block of bone that was trapezoidal in shape was resected. This piece consisted of glabellar, ethmoidal, and nasal bones. The ethmoid cells were exenterated. In addition, parts of the septum and turbinates were removed in order to create room for the medial translocation of the orbitonasal complex and to maintain an adequate airway as well.

Lateral and inferior orbital wall osteotomies, as described previously, were performed. From the midline surgical defect of the anterior cranial base, the osteotomy was made across the roof of the orbits to connect with the cuts made on the lateral orbital walls. The anterior halves of the orbits were totally detached.

Tears in the nasal mucosa were repaired with chromic sutures. The mobilized anterior segment of each orbit was brought to the midline, wired to the other, and their superior margins transfixed to the frontal bandeau that served as the guide for their alignment, as well as a stable bar on which they were suspended. The nasal bones were also wired together, incorporating a bone graft in the mid-dorsum to rebuild the nasal bridge. Trimming the margins of the pyriform aperture enlarged the choanal opening that had become narrowed after medially shifting the nasal bones. The alar cartilages were brought together over the tip of the bone graft to correct the bifid nasal lobule. Medial canthopexies were performed. Finally, the widely separated eyebrows moved nearer to each other after a midline resection of redundant skin of the forehead and nose (Fig. 6–3C).

Hypotelorism

When the interorbital distance is less than 30 mm in an adult, the eyes appear hypoteloric,

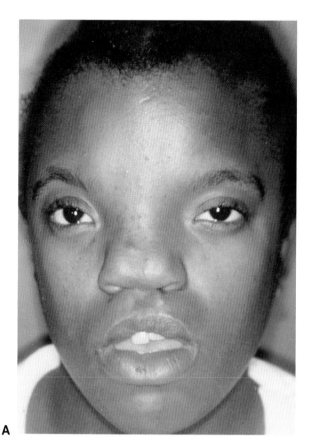

A

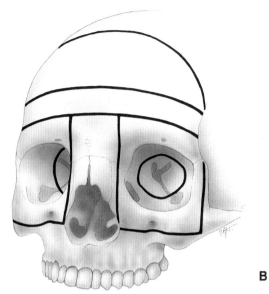

B

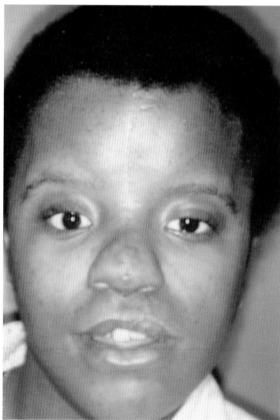

C

Figure 6–3.   **A:** A case of severe hypertelorism with side-set eyes and bifid nasal bridge. **B:** Outline of the osteotomies performed to allow movements of the orbits medially and correction of the bifid nose. **C:** Postoperative appearance at 3 years.

or close together. Visual disturbances are rare. A mongoloid slant of the palpebral fissure is commonly present. Premature fusion of the metopic sutures results in narrowing of the forehead and is generally associated with close-set eyes. In mild cases, expectant treatment has resulted in some improvement. Surgery is directed primarily toward recontouring the frontal bone deformity. Hypotelorism in the presence of a medial cleft of the lip is commonly associated with prosencephaly and bears a grave prognosis.

Orbital Dystopia

An anomalous position of the orbits is referred to as orbital dystopia. Since the term "hyperteleorbitism" has long been adopted for lateral displacement, dystopia is the designation for positional deviations in a vertical orientation. Like hyperteleorbitism, it is not an autonomous condition, but rather a manifestation related to certain anomalies or syndromes. These include unilateral orbitofacial clefts, unilateral craniosynostosis, craniofacial dysostosis, and tumors.

Congenital dystopia, which accompanies plagiocephaly, may remain stationary or sometimes show improvement with growth. In contrast, dystopia in orbitofacial clefts tends to get worse. Preferably, defects of the orbit and maxilla are bone grafted preliminary to the translocation of the orbit and globe. Elevation of the orbit necessitates a frontal craniotomy and the creation of a hemicoronal bandeau. Osteotomies of the four walls of the affected orbit are performed. A segment of bone from its upper margin is removed. This should create a space to give room for the orbit to be elevated to a level matching the normal side. The piece of bone removed is transferred as a graft to the gap in the maxilla.[13,14]

An inferior displacement of the orbit can also be achieved by reversing the site of removal of the strip of bone, i.e., from the inferior margin of the orbit; this is used to graft the gap in the forehead. An alternate method may be performed extracranially by a U-shaped osteotomy of the socket. This is demonstrated in Figure 6–4. The caudal part of the mobilized unit was not removed, but was overlapped on the maxilla

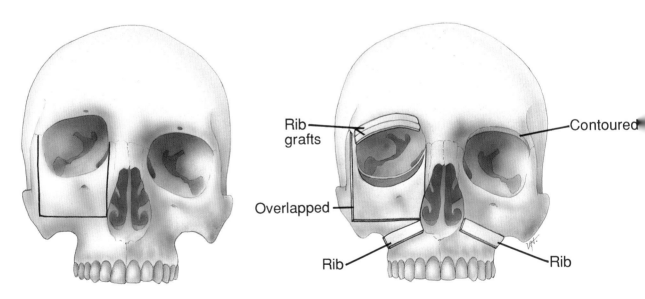

Figure 6–4. Outline of a case with a right orbital dystopia. The diagram on the left outlines the osteotomy, and the diagram on the right shows the repositioned orbital segment and the rib grafts in place.

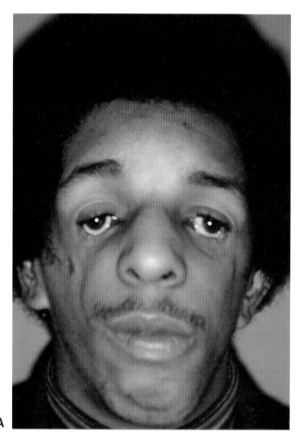

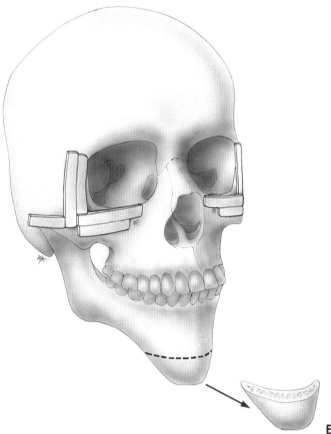

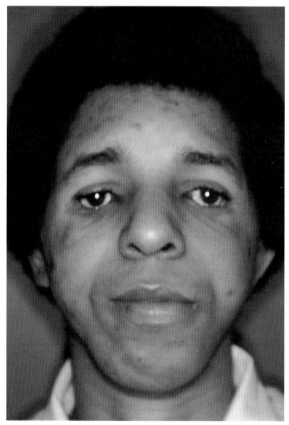

Figure 6–5. A: A case of Treacher Collins syndrome with all the classic facial features, including lack of malar prominence, downslanted palpebral fissures, eyelid colobomas, and a retrodisplaced chin protruberance. **B:** Outline of the reconstruction about the orbits and zygomas with rib grafts. A sliding genioplasty with a rib over graft was also performed. **C:** Patient's postoperative appearance 3 years after a rhinoplasty and dermafat-free grafts to the cheeks.

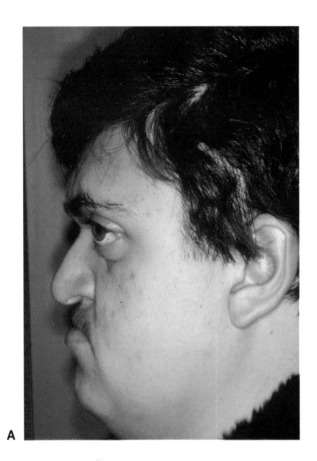

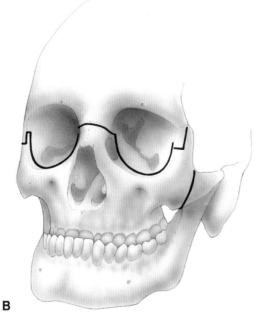

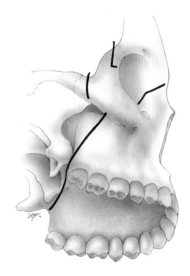

Figure 6–6. **A:** A typical example of a Crouzon syndrome, which has the prominent eyes, midface hypoplasia, retrusion of the maxilla. **B:** Outline of the osteotomies done in a LeFort III type for a midface advancement. The details are discussed more fully in the text. *(Figure Continues.)*

Figure 6–6 *(continued).* **C:** A postoperative view after the surgery with a LeFort III advancement completed. The dental malocclusion was improved and the midface was brought into a more normal contour.

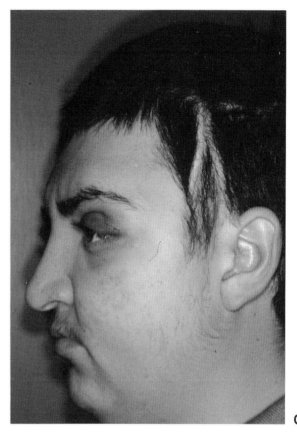

c

to give some fullness to the somewhat flattened cheek on the affected side. Rib grafts were inserted beneath the roof of the orbit to obliterate the dead space that was formed after the globe descended. The undetached medial ligament also moved downward and caused the lid fissure to be in line with its counterpart on the opposite side.

Orbital Clefts

Clefts of the orbit are extremely rare, compared with clefts of the lip and palate. These unusual entities occur most often in conjunction with other forms of facial clefts. The orbital cleft most frequently encountered is associated with mandibulofacial dysostosis, or Treacher Collins syndrome. It is due to hypoplasia of the malar bone, the main component of the inferolateral segment of the orbital wall. In its most severe expression, the zygoma is totally missing. Consequently, the lateral portion of the supraorbital ridge is depressed, transforming the plane of the orbit from horizontal to oblique, and the palpebral opening assumes an antimongoloid slant.

There is also a deficiency of lower lid substance characterized by a coloboma or notching and absence of lashes at the medial lid margin. The nose is prominent, the maxilla narrow, and an antegonal notch is present at the body of the mandible. Microtia of varying severity is common. The upper airway in young patients is invariably narrow, making airway management difficult during intubation.

The aim of surgery for Treacher Collins syndrome is primarily to correct the eyelid defect and to position the eyelid and reconstruct the deficiency of the bony orbit. Secondarily, it is to improve the facial aesthetics (rhinoplasty, orthognathic surgery, etc.) The patient in Figure 6–5A is a 22-year-old man with Treacher Collins syndrome.

The orbits were exposed through a bicoronal scalp incision that extended to the front of the tragi. Bilateral lower lid incisions gave additional exposure to the maxillae and orbital floors. The downslanted superolateral orbital rims were burred to reshape the lateral corners of the roofs. Split ribs were used to build the floors, lateral walls, and infraorbital rims (Fig.

6–5B). The zygomatic arches were constructed with additional rib grafts wedged into the temporal bones. The lateral canthi were elevated and the lower lid skin augmented with transposed upper lid skin flaps.

Subsequent operations included a chin advancement, a corrective rhinoplasty, Z-plasties to transpose the sideburns, and dermafat-free grafts to fill in the hollow of the cheeks (Fig. 6–5C).

Craniofacial Dysostosis

Generic usage of the term includes several related or interrelated malformations (Crouzon, Apert, Pfeiffer, Chotzen-Saethre, Carpenter) where both cranial and facial involvement are usually present. Crouzon is considered the most common. The classic description emphasizes the triad of cranial deformity, midfacial hypoplasia, and occular exorbitism.

Phenotypically, these diverse craniofacial syndromes have salient features that identify them separately. However, wide variations occur in their clinical expressions. In some instances, one syndrome seems to merge into the other. This problem does not alter surgical decisions, since the same principles in reconstruction apply to virtually all forms.

Cranial Deformity

Secondary deformities occur in the calvarium as a consequence of early fusion or synostosis of the cranial sutures. The cranial base may be involved as well. The operations for the calvarial component in craniofacial dysostosis are discussed in Chapter 5.

Midface Hypoplasia

Retromaxillism or midface retrusion is a salient feature of craniofacial dysostosis (Fig. 6–6A). The maxilla is not only retruded, but it may be poorly developed in both anteroposterior and superoinferior directions, as frequently observed in Apert syndrome. In the most severe presentation, hypoplasia occurs in three dimensions. There is dental crowding with narrowing of the maxillary arch. The jaw juts forward more obviously in a class III malocclusion, usually with an open bite. The deep vault of the palate is lined with a thickened mucoperiosteum that may form as heavy folds along the lingual sides of the alveolus, creating a midline depression or pseudocleft.

The surgical objectives for midface hypoplasia are to increase orbital depth, project the midface, and bring the teeth into good occlusion. After a midface advancement, an increment in nasopharyngeal space enhances airflow and improves voice resonance in patients with denasality.

A standard operation for the typical patient with Crouzon's disease is craniofacial dysjunction by osteotomies of the LeFort III type or its modifications (Fig. 6–6).

A bicoronal scalp incision gives wide exposure of the orbits, nose, and subtemporal fossae with direct access to the retromolar areas. Osteotomies are made across the frontonasal juncture and medial walls of the orbits above the lachrimal crests. These are then continued to the floors and lateral walls, as described previously for exorbitism. The external cut on the lateral orbital walls is extended inferiorly around the maxillary tubercles to the pterygomaxillary fissures. Through intraoral incisions, pterygomaxillary separation is induced with a curved osteotome. Having done this on both sides, the midfacial block is detached after severance of the nose from the septovomerine connection through the nasofrontal gap, without disturbing the endotracheal tube. The midface is then disimpacted, mobilized, and advanced forward in a slightly downward direction. This movement causes some elongation at the middle third of the face and derotates the mandible. The open gaps at key osteotomy sites are bone grafted. The upper and lower teeth are wired in occlusion, and the maxilla is immobilized with suspension wires to the cranium.

Although the LeFort III osteotomy is best suited for craniofacial dysostosis, patients with the typical triad of deformities and patients with atypical malformations may require a modified approach to treatment. An example was a 19-year-old woman who had undergone a long course of orthodontic therapy (Fig. 6–7). She rejected the recommendation for a midface advancement with orthognathic surgery, since she did not wish to be encumbered with her teeth wired together for several weeks. Instead, she accepted an orbitonasal advancement for her

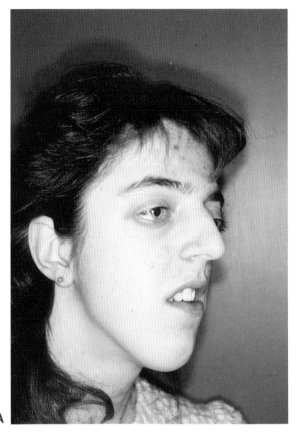
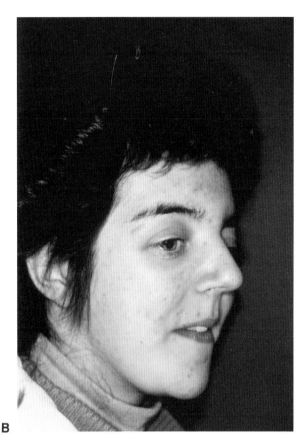

A

B

Figure 6-7. **A:** A Crouzon syndrome associated with a long face deformity. **B:** Postoperative appearance at 7 months.

mild exorbitism. Her long face appearance was made more acceptable by a vertical reduction of chin height and an advancement genioplasty. A reduction rhinoplasty was also performed.

The LeFort II osteotomy is appropriate for nasomaxillary retrusion with a class III malocclusion and the zygomas appearing normal (Fig. 6-8). The usual line of osteotomy is started from the nasofrontal area and is diverted inferiorly past the lachrimal fossa. From the orbital floor, it is directed anteriorly across the orbital rim just medial to the orbital foramen and proceeds inferolaterally below the zygomatic buttress toward the maxillary tuberosity. The maxilla is cleaved from the pterygoid plates in the same manner as described during a LeFort III osteotomy. The opposite side is treated similarly. After completion of the osteotomies, the midface segment is moved forward, teeth placed in occlusion and wired, bone grafts inserted, and immobilization established similar to that rendered for the LeFort III operation.

A LeFort I osteotomy is commonly employed during orthognathic surgery to restore a normal occlusal relationship of the maxilla to the mandible (Fig. 6-9). A horizontal cut is made above the apices of the teeth from the pyriform aperture to the maxillopterygoid fissure on both sides. In asymmetric deformities, segmental osteotomies are done so that affected parts are free to be moved and fixed in a more desirable position. Stabilization of these segments is attained by bone grafts, interosseous wirings, or, more recently, with the use of miniplates.

A review of these techniques and an understanding of the various approaches will offer the neurosurgeon and craniofacial team a number of different strategies in approaching the midface, orbits, and the skull base. This chapter is designed as an adjunct to Chapter 7, which deals especially with tumors of the skull base and intracranial regions. These surgical approaches are always a multiteam approach involving neurosurgeons, plastic surgeons, maxil-

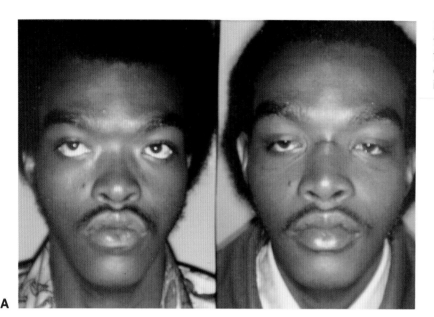

A

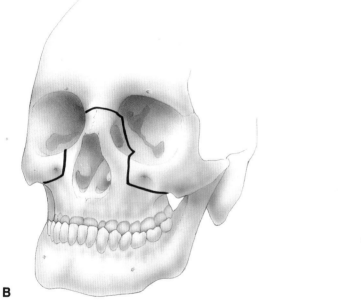

B

Figure 6–8.   **A:** A case of retrusion of the central portion of the middle third of the face. **B:** Outline of the LeFort II type of osteotomy performed to correct this maxillary retrusion. *(Figure Continues.)*

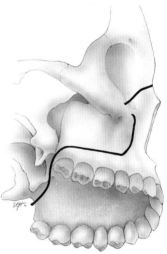

Figure 6–8 *(continued).*   **C:** Preoperative appearance and postoperative appearance at 8 months.

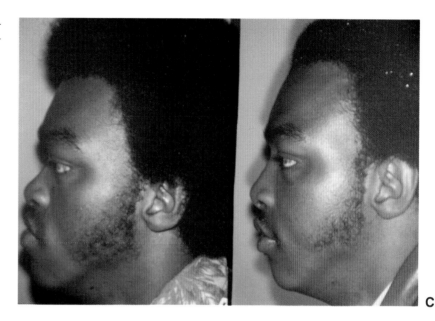

C

lofacial and oral surgeons. This team approach allows for some very sophisticated and quite complex neurosurgical adventures.

References

1. Tessier P. Osteotomies totales de la face, syndrome de Crouzon, syndrome D'Apert, oxycephalies, turricephalies. Ann Chir Plast 1967;12:273–86.
2. McCarthy JG. LeFort III advancement osteotomy in the growing child. In: Carone EP (ed). Craniofacial Surgery. Boston: Little Brown, 1985:123–33.
3. Tessier P. Apert's syndrome: Acrocephalosyndactyly types. In: Carone EP (ed). Craniofacial Surgery. Boston: Little Brown, 1985:280–303.
4. Ortiz-Monasterio F, Fuente del Campo A, Carrillo A. Advancement of the orbits and the midface in one piece, combined with frontal repositioning, for the correction of Crouzon deformities. Plast Reconstr Surg 1978;61:507–16.
5. Whitaker LA, Munro IR, Salyer KE, Jackson IT, Ortiz-Monasterio F, Marchac D. Combined report on problems and complications in 793 craniofacial operations. Plast Reconstr Surg 1979;64:198–203.
6. David JD, Poswillo P, Simpson D. Craniosynostosis: Causes, Natural History, and Management. Berlin: Springer-Verlag, 1982:283–8.
7. Lewin ML, Argamaso RV. Midface osteotomies for correction of facial deformities (craniofacial dysos-

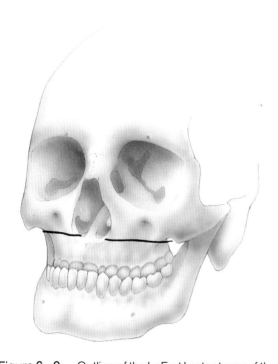

Figure 6–9.   Outline of the LeFort I osteotomy of the maxilla.

tosis and maxillary hypoplasia). Trans Am Acad Ophthalmol Otolaryngol 1972;76:946–55.

8. Tessier P, Guiot G, Rougerie J, Delbet JP, Pastoriza J. Osteotomies cranio-naso-orbito-faciales, hypertelorisme. Ann Chir Plast 1967;12:103–18.

9. Tessier P. Experiences in the treatment of orbital hypertelorism. Plast Reconstr Surg 1974;53:1–18.

10. Edgerton MT, Udavarhelyi GB, Knox DL. The surgical correction of occular hypertelorism. Ann Surg 1970;172:473–96.

11. Converse JM, Ransohoff J, Mathews ES, Smith B, Molenar A. Occular hypertelorism and pseudohypertelorism: Advances in surgical treatment. Plast Reconstr Surg 1970;45:1–13.

12. Psillakis JM. Surgical treatment of hypertelorism. In: Carone EP (ed). Craniofacial Surgery. Boston: Little Brown, 1985:190–9.

13. Edgerton MY, Jane JA. Vertical dystopia—surgical correction. Plast Reconstr Surg 1981;67:121–38.

14. Furnas DW, Achauer BM. Two cases of orbital dystopia: Tessier III cleft and craniofacial osteotomas. Ann Plast Surg 1981;6:66–70.

SEVEN

Kalmon D. Post, M.D.
Andrew Blitzer, M.D.

Surgery of the Skull Base

Because of its technical complexies, cranial base surgery was eliminated from consideration as a therapeutic option until relatively recently. This exclusion was equally true for benign and malignant disease. While early reports demonstrated the feasibility of craniofacial surgery, they also noted the high morbidity and mortality, particularly from cerebrospinal fluid (CSF) leakage and infection.[1,2]

However, as operative frontiers were conquered, previously inaccessible areas such as the cavernous sinus, superior orbital fissures, infratemporal fossae, clivus, and temporal bone all became available to surgery.[3]

It is clear that cranial base surgery is a multidisciplinary undertaking involving neurosurgeons, otolaryngology/head and neck surgeons, and plastic surgeons. Sophisticated imaging is mandatory to define the extent of disease and its relationship to surrounding normal structures. Computed tomography (CT) scan with bone algorithms, magnetic resonance imaging (MRI), and angiography are all of vital importance. Recent dynamic studies of the internal carotid artery with subsequent xenon cerebral blood flow studies allow determination of whether the carotid artery can be resected without reconstruction.[4,5]

The anatomy of the cranial base permits division into the anterior, middle, and posterior fossae with their corresponding anatomical limits, contents, and extracranial structures. Despite these distinctions, some tumors will cross these regions and share features and surgical considerations.

Several factors must be considered, including the biologic and anatomical nature of the tumor, the ability to resect while preserving neurologic function, and cosmetic deformities. Sacrificing some neurologic function such as unilateral vision or hearing is often the difficult course of choice when survival is at stake. With ethmoid and maxillary sinus carcinoma, the orbit will be involved more than 50% of the time and will require exenteration with the tumor mass.

The general objectives will be: good visualization, complete tumor removal, sparing of neural function, and acceptable cosmetic deformities.

Craniofacial Resection for Anterior Skull Base Tumors

Cancers of the paranasal sinuses tend to have a poor prognosis. They have an insidious onset, follow a protracted clinical course, and are poorly controlled by most forms of therapy. Their diagnosis is often delayed, and patient survival is compromised by direct extension of the tumor into the cranial cavity and orbit, as well as into such surgically inaccessible sites as the retropharyngeal nodes.

All of the paranasal sinuses except the maxillary sinus have a common wall with the cranial cavity. Their proximity to the cranial cavity has hindered the kind of en bloc tumor resection done in the inferiorly located maxillary sinus. Consequently, conservative surgery in these sinuses is fraught with local recurrence at the cribriform plate and base of the skull. The exceedingly poor survival rate, 8% overall at 5 years, is caused primarily by uncontrolled local disease, with only 10% dying as a result of metastases.[6,7]

The relative safety and propriety of the combined craniofacial resection was well established by the work of Ketcham et al.[1] In 1963, they evaluated the results obtained in a study of 30 patients with advanced paranasal sinus, nasal and orbital cancers treated at the National Institutes of Health, mostly failures of other treatment modalities. After careful evaluation, 19 of these patients were found to be candidates for combined resection. With the exception of one perioperative mortality related to infection, these patients did well. In 1968, Ketcham and coworkers reviewed their 10-year experience, reporting a cure rate of approximately 30% in an otherwise unsalvageable group of patients.[2] By 1973, the cure rate rose to a 50% determinate 5-year survival.[6]

Development of reconstructive surgery for craniofacial malformations added to the advancement of the craniofacial resection technique.[8,9] New modifications were made as surgeons embraced Ketcham's work. In 1975, Westbury and associates[10] reported using a frontal sinus osteoplastic flap as an approach for combined resection. Sisson et al.[11] expanded on Ketcham's work via a frontal craniotomy and described methods of skull base reconstruction employing bone and cartilage. Shah and Galicich[12] strongly recommended the use of a bi-frontal craniotomy because it provided additional exposure, permitted better assessment of tumor resectability and facilitated dural resection and repair. Schramm et al.,[13] in 1979, expanded the role of the frontal burr hole and described the use of a frontotemporal flap for cases with greater involvement of the skull base.

Indications

The combined craniofacial resection is indicated in patients who are good surgical risks and who have malignant tumors of the superior nasal cavity, ethmoid sinus (see Fig. 7–7A), frontal sinus, and orbit. This combined technique has also been employed for benign, but locally aggressive, tumors of this region, such as esthesioneuroblastomas[14,15] (see Fig. 7–9), meningiomas, fibro-osseous lesions,[16] chordomas and osteomas. Juvenile angiofibromas with intracranial extension also can be managed with this approach.[17]

Patients with systemic diseases who are in poor condition or have metastases are not candidates for craniofacial resection. CT or MRI demonstration of involvement of the nasopharynx, superior and posterior sphenoid or sphenoid ridge, invasion at the optic chiasm, prevertebral space extension, or significant intracranial or intracerebral extension contraindicates these procedures.

Usually, combined craniofacial resection has been reserved for tumors that appear resectable. If there is significant intracranial intradural extension, aggressive surgery has been excluded. However, palliation of disease should be an important consideration. If intractable pain or a large fungating mass is present, surgery may be performed to alleviate these problems and promote a better quality of survival.[17]

Craniofacial surgery is done most commonly to expose the midline and paramedian structures, including the cribriform plate, ethmoid sinuses with medial walls of the orbits, and the anterior wall of the sphenoid sinus (Fig. 7–1).[18] The limitations of resection include involvement of the optic chiasm and cavernous sinus superiorly and the carotid canal inferiorly.

Preoperative Evaluation

Radiographic examination should include standard sinus x-rays, including a submental vertex

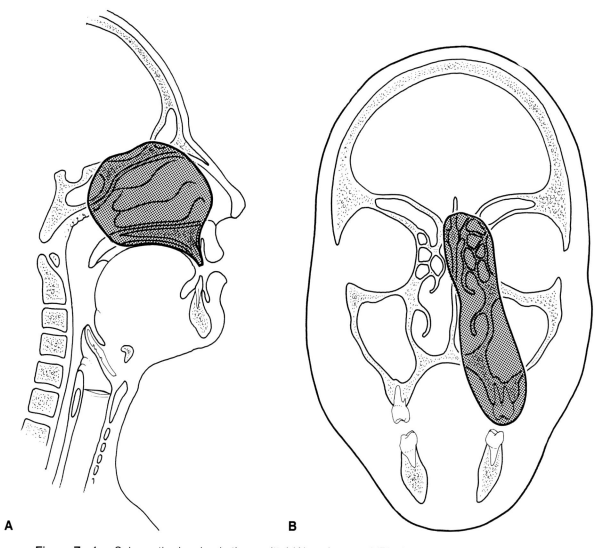

Figure 7 – 1. Schematic drawing in the sagittal (A) and coronal (B) planes demonstrating the areas of surgical resection.

projection, to detect erosion of the lesser wing of the sphenoid and middle cranial fossa extension. Clouding of the sphenoid should not contraindicate surgery, since this condition may be inflammatory in nature.

Tomography of the skull base is also useful for evaluating erosion of the sphenoid bone. Angiography may demonstrate the invasion, compression, or displacement of the carotid artery or jugular venous system. It will also give information regarding the vascularity of the tumor and demonstrate major feeding vessels. Embolization of feeding arteries may be considered in order to make subsequent surgery easier and safer.

The CT scan with bone algorithms and the MRI with gadolinium enhancement are excel-lent for evaluating the extent of the lesion. They show dural or intracranial involvement, displacement or invasion of orbital structures, and cavernous sinus encroachment, as well as bony integrity. Axial, sagittal, and coronal projections are needed for surgical decisions. (Figs. 7 – 7B, 7 – 9A – D).

Techniques

Airway compromise is uncommon in midface cancer resection, making a preliminary tracheostomy rarely necessary.

The surgical approach consists of a bifrontal intracranial neurosurgical exposure combined with a transfacial exposure performed by ear, nose, and throat (ENT). Following the induction

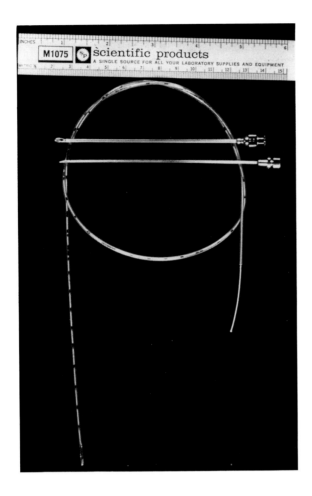

Figure 7–2. Spinal drainage is established using a 5 F Stamey ureteral catheter passed through a 14 gauge Tuohy needle. A blunt end no. 20 needle is connected to the catheter and a closed collection system attached.[19]

of general anesthesia, a lumbar subarachnoid drain is placed and used intraoperatively and for 3 to 5 days postoperatively to drain the CSF (Fig. 7–2).[19]

A bicoronal scalp flap with a bifrontal bone flap has been used in most of our cases (Fig. 7–3). A unilateral exposure is indicated for asymmetrical benign disease, orbital disease, or other lateral processes. The flap is based inferiorly on supraorbital and supratrochlear vessels, and laterally on branches of the superficial temporal arteries.

The pericranium is elevated bifrontally in all cases, leaving intact the frontal base attachment with the blood supply (Figs. 7–4, 7–7C).

A free bifrontal bone flap is cut and elevated (Fig. 7–7D). Once the bone flap is removed, cerebral decompression to allow blunt dissection of the dura is achieved by removing 20 to 60 ml of CSF through the spinal drainage system and administering mannitol (Table 7–1). An epidural dissection along the floor is carried

back to the planum. In the region of the cribriform plate, the olfactory nerves with their dural sleeves must be cut. To prevent a CSF leak, each small hole is closed immediately with a 4-0 silk suture (Figs. 7–7E, 7–9G).

Wide intracranial exposure has been used along with lumbar spinal drainage to minimize frontal lobe retraction. This allows exposure of the skull base and dura as far posteriorly as the tuberculum sella and sphenoid wings. Intradural exposure is obtained if the basal dura is invaded by tumor (Fig. 7–9G). The wide basal exposure offers several advantages (Table 7–2). Skull base cuts can be easily varied as dictated by the pathologic anatomy (Figs. 7–5, 7–7E). When dura is involved, suturing of dural patch

Table 7–1.   Adjuncts to Cranial Base Surgery

Spinal drainage for 3 to 5 days
Mannitol
Prophylactic antibiotics

Figure 7 – 3. Drawing depicting the bicoronal scalp flap and a modified Weber-Ferguson lateral rhinotomy incision, with or without lip splitting.

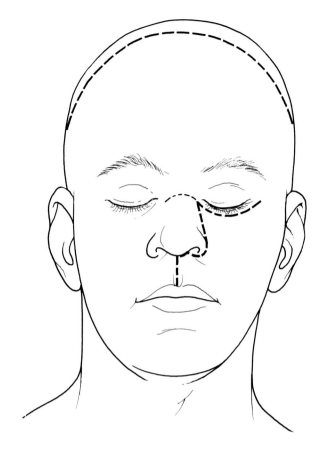

Figure 7 – 4. Schematic drawing demonstrating the periosteal flap based along the frontal ridge leaving the blood supply intact.

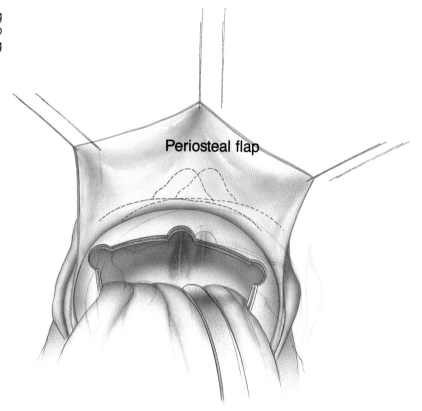

Table 7–2. Advantages of Combined
Craniofacial Resection

1. Wide exposure
2. Accurate evaulation of intracranial extension
3. Protection of brain
4. Intradural and extradural access
5. Ease of dural replacement
6. Security of dural closure
7. Facilitates en bloc resection
8. Adaptable
9. Cosmetically acceptable

grafts is facilitated (Fig. 7–9G). Transcranial facial dissection is also made easier by wide exposures and base resection.

If the tumor is resectable, the area of the skull base removal is outlined with a high speed drill and osteotome (Fig. 7–7E). This process should include the ipsilateral ethmoid labyrinth, superior and lateral walls of the sphenoid, anterior cranial fossa, and the cribriform plate. The resection can be extended to include the orbital roof, opposite ethmoid, or the frontal sinus (see Fig. 7–7I). The facial incision is usually a modified Weber-Ferguson lateral rhinotomy, with or without lip splitting (Figs. 7–3, 7–7F, 7–9E, F). Midline face splitting and degloving procedures have also been recommended. After the facial dissection is completed, the brain is retracted again and, working from above and below, the entire specimen is delivered through the facial opening (Fig. 7–7G, H).

Following the completed resection and specimen removal, repair of the anterior cranial fossa is begun, utilizing the pericranial flap raised at the beginning of the procedure. The pericranium is draped over the defect and the remaining floor of the anterior cranial fossa. It is sutured to the dura inferiorly to keep it in position and allow it to act as a sling for the frontal lobes (Fig. 7–6).

The technique of dural patch and periosteal sling suturing is most important to prevent CSF leakage. A frontal periosteum sling is brought beneath the frontal lobes and is sutured to the

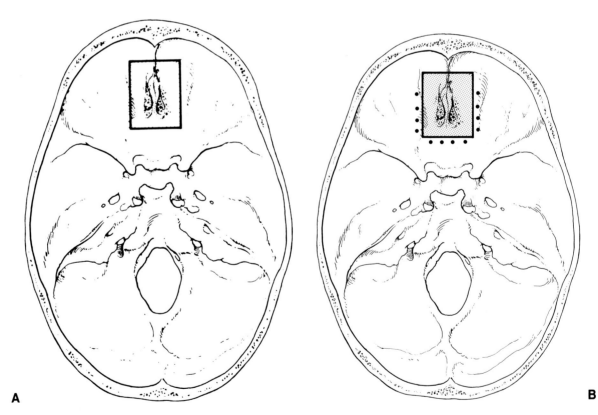

A   B

Figure 7–5.   **A**: Schematic drawing of the skull base outlining the anterior region to be resected.
B: Schematic drawing demonstrating the holes drilled along the edge of the bone defect to facilitate periosteal sutures.

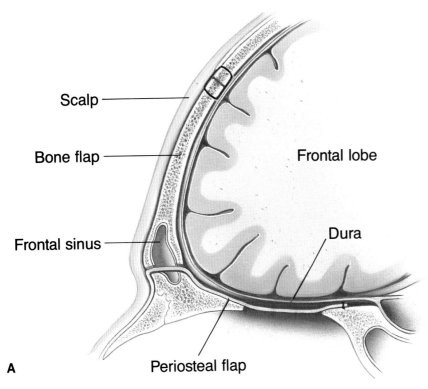

Scalp

Bone flap

Frontal lobe

Frontal sinus

Dura

Periosteal flap

A

Figure 7-6. **A**: Drawing depicting the midline sagittal plane with the periosteal flap rotated beneath the frontal dura, across the bone defect, and sutured to the dura at the level of the planum. This periosteal flap supports the frontal lobes. **B**. Drawing depicting a more lateral sagittal plane with the periosteal flap sutured to the holes in the bone edge, as well as to the dura. *(Figure Continues.)*

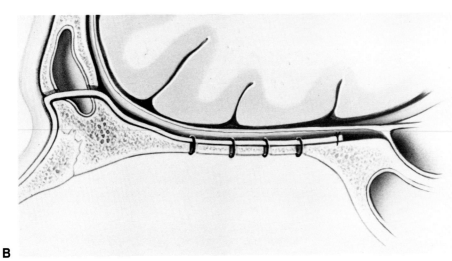

B

basal dura over the posterior planum (Fig. 7-6). The periosteal flap is also sutured to the edges of the skull base resection. This has been facilitated by drilling holes for additional sutures along the resected edge (Fig. 7-5B) to be certain the periosteal flap covers the entire opening in the skull base without slipping forward. The sutures are placed through the facial opening. Galeofrontalis flaps, which receive blood from the supraorbital, supratrochlear, and superficial temporal arteries, are stronger because they are thicker and may be preferred.[3] However, since they cause the scalp to be thin and devascularized, they are not used by our group. Regional myo-

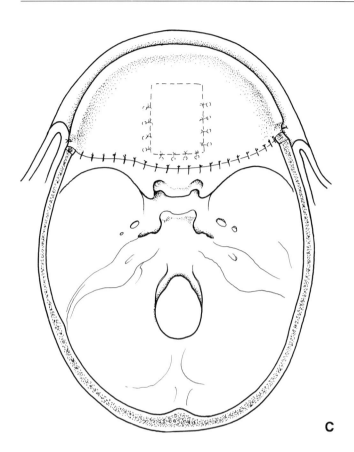

Figure 7 – 6 *(continued)*.   **C**: Drawing depicting skull base with periosteal flap sutured beneath the frontal lobes to the bone edge and the dura.

c

cutaneous flaps or distant microvascular pedicled muscle grafts attached to the superficial artery and vein have been utilized.[20-22] These have been necessary for large defects and in one instance of postoperative infection which threatened the exposed dura through the sinuses. The latissimus dorsi muscle is the most commonly used (Fig. 7–8).

The dura is then returned to its original position, and further tacking sutures are used to attach the dura to the pericranial flap near the superoanterior surface. We generally have not needed any other materials for skull base reconstruction, although occasionally we have used screen mesh. Osseous reconstruction of the surgical defect is necessary only when the tumor invades the craniofacial skeleton. Autogenous bone graft or alloplastic materials may be used. Bony reconstruction is done if there is a contour defect of the anterior or superior calvarium. A split-thickness skin graft is placed over the pericranium and held in place with a bolus of Xeroform gauze (Fig. 7–7J); the remaining facial incisions are closed (Fig. 7–7K, L, M). If there is a palatal defect, a surgical stent is inserted and

wired into position. Occasionally, reconstruction of the nose is required. Bone from the inner table of the calvarium is wired in position.

Complications

Infection and CSF leak are the most common complications of craniofacial surgery. The incidence is higher in patients who have received preoperative radiotherapy. The cases in which the dura is resected have the highest possibility of leak, and the best solution is prevention by meticulous intraoperative dural closure.

Using this technique, we have had no CSF leaks or meningitis, and the only complications have been two delayed bone flap infections. The cosmetic results have been excellent, requiring only the use of an eye patch if orbital exenteration is necessary (Figs. 7–7K, L, M, 7–9H, I).

Even if cure is not achieved, the craniofacial resection yields excellent pain relief. We therefore advise this procedure in most anterior skull base tumors in view of the significant benefit and extremely low complication rate.

Figure 7–7.   **A**: A 57-year-old man developed severe facial pain and mild proptosis. Lateral and frontal tomograms demonstrate a mass (arrows) in the ethmoid sinus. **B**: Axial (top) and coronal (bottom) enhanced CT scan demonstrating an undifferentiated carcinoma (arrow) in the ethmoid sinus and orbit. *(Figure Continues.)*

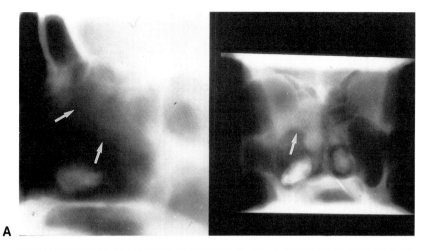

A

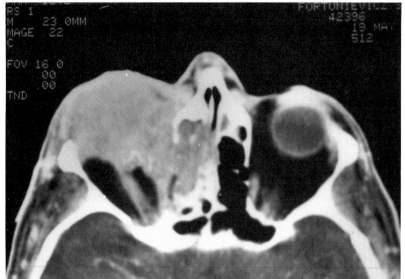

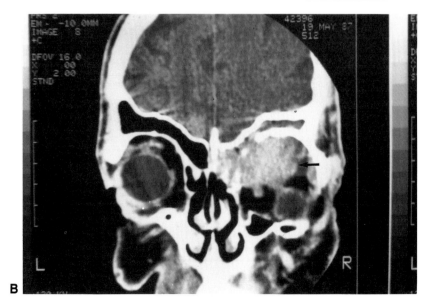

B

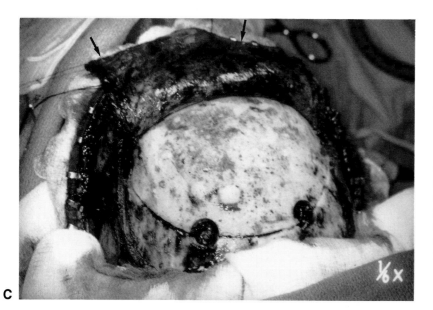

C

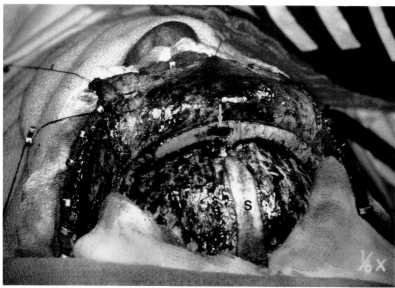

D

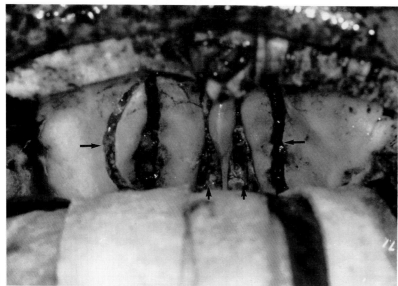

E

Figure 7–7 *(continued)*. C: Intraoperative view of the scalp flap, periosteal flap (arrows), and bifrontal craniotomy cuts. **D:** The bone flap has been elevated. The frontal sinus has been crossed (arrow), and the superior sagittal sinus (S) protected with Gelfoam. **E:** The dura has been elevated off the frontal floor and protected with cottonoids. The olfactory nerves have been transsected and the dural sleeves have been cut and sutured closed. The olfactory grooves are well seen (arrowheads). The cuts in the base are evident (arrows). Note that the initial cut on the left side was not lateral enough to pass the tumor; therefore a second cut was made. *(Figure Continues.)*

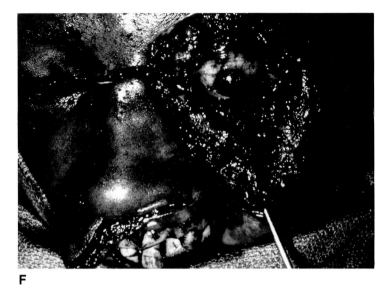

F

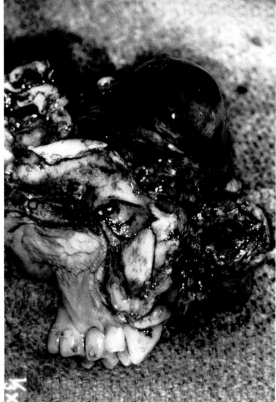

G

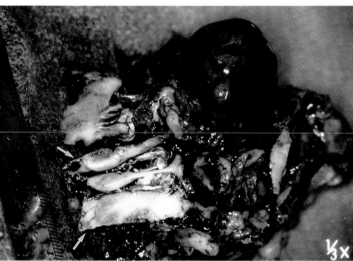

H

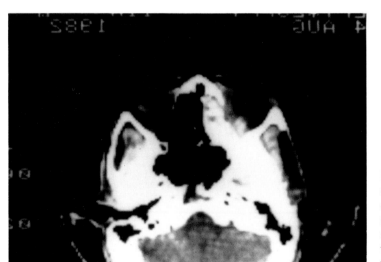

I

Figure 7–7 *(continued).* **F**: The facial incision and early dissection have begun. The left orbit will be exenterated. **G**: Lateral view of the en bloc resected specimen. **H**: Superior view of the en bloc resected specimen. Note the cribriform plate (arrows) still attached. **I**: Axial CT scan showing the extent of resection. *(Figure Continues.)*

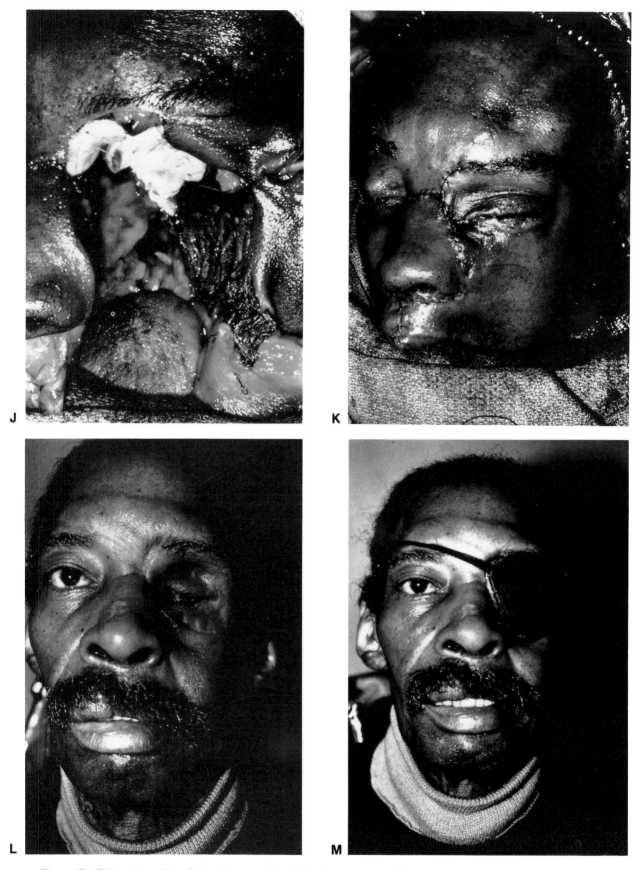

Figure 7-7 *(continued)*.   **J**: Xeroform packing following resection. **K, L, M:** Cosmetic result following resection. The patient preferred only an eye patch.

136

Figure 7–8. Intraoperative bifrontal view demonstrating a latissimus dorsi muscle transfer graft filling the subfrontal and anterior defect. Note the superficial temporal artery and vein anastamoses (arrow).

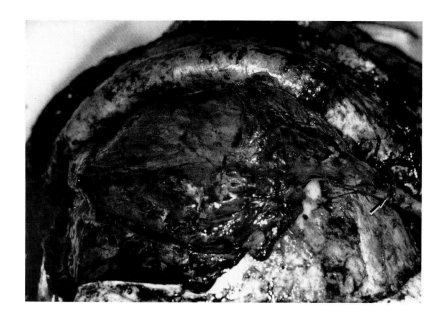

Anterolateral Skull Base Tumors

Meningiomas in the sphenoid wing and cavernous sinus comprise the largest group of anterolateral skull base tumors. However, chordomas, chondrosarcomas, and adenoid cystic carcinomas also are amenable to this approach.

Intracavernous meningiomas recently have been removed aggressively by some teams,[23–25] but until now we have relied on radiation treatment more than open resection.[26,27] In our judgment the potential deficits due to intracavernous manipulation have outweighed the possible benefits. Nevertheless, if visual function has been lost, or in the presence of very aggressive disease, such as adenoid cystic carcinoma, we have considered more vigorous surgery, including potential resection of the cavernous sinus and bypassing of the carotid.

The circulation is studied with angiography on admission, and if necessary because of insufficient collaterals, an extracranial to intracranial bypass procedure is done to eliminate the need for the internal carotid.

At surgery, the exposure is obtained through a bifrontal craniotomy with unilateral temporal extension. The orbital roof and lateral wall are removed via osteotomies. The zygoma and temporomandibular joint are mobilized, exposing the trigeminal nerve, the internal carotid artery, the cavernous sinus, and the optic nerves. Then aggressive resection of the anterolateral skull base can be performed sacrificing the cavernous sinus region if necessary. With benign disease, the procedure must be modified according to the patient's age, function, and medical status.

The main difficulty occurs in sealing the dura and eliminating a CSF leak. The dura must be meticulously reconstructed, often using pericranial or temporalis fascia. If possible, a vascularized pedicled flap is rotated.

At times, it may be necessary for a two-stage procedure with intradural resection and closure first, followed by extradural tumor and bone resection with reconstruction at a later date. The reconstruction requires separating the dural, neural, and vascular structures from the sinuses and pharyngeal mucosa. Both frontal and temporal periosteal flaps are utilized, as well as muscular flaps, for which either the temporalis muscle or a microvascular transfer of the latissimus is very common. The lateral bone is replaced securely for cosmetic reconstruction.

Middle Cranial Base

The temporal bone and its relationships make up the majority of the middle cranial base. The internal carotid artery passes through the temporal bone to get from extracranial to intracranial. Major venous structures, including the transverse sinus, sigmoid sinus, and petrosal sinuses also are involved with the temporal bone.

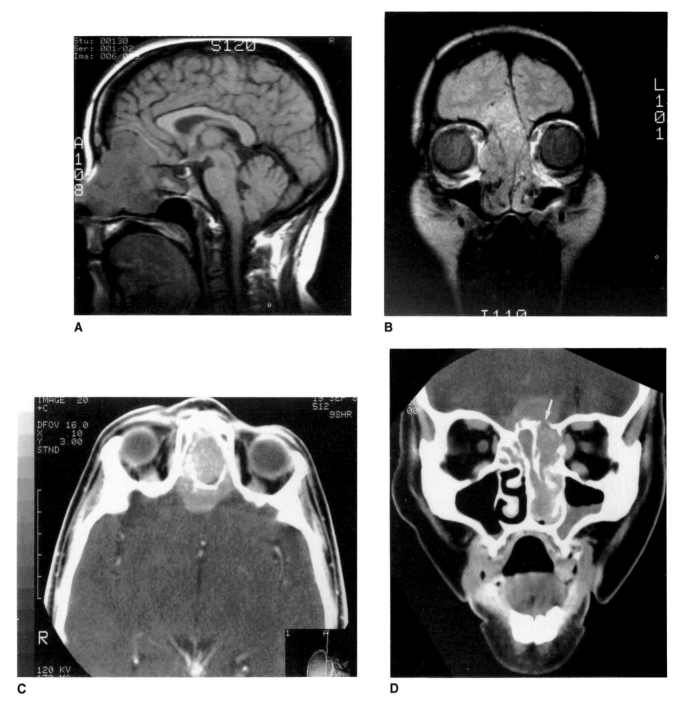

A

B

C

D

Figure 7–9.   **A**: A 41-year-old woman had a history of epistaxis and a mass in the right nasal cavity. Biopsy showed esthesioneuroblastoma. Thereafter she received 5400 rads over 47 days. Subsequently, MRI scans failed to show shrinkage. CSF rhinorrhea developed and she presented with pneumococcal meningitis. Sagittal MRI demonstrating a large subfrontal and intranasal esthesioneuroblastoma. It has extended through the dura on the right side. **B**: Coronal MRI demonstrating the same tumor. The orbital contents have not been invaded. **C**: Axial enhanced CT scan demonstrating the tumor through the cribriform plate. **D**: Coronal enhanced CT scan showing the tumor and the bone destruction at the right cribriform plate (arrow). *(Figure Continues.)*

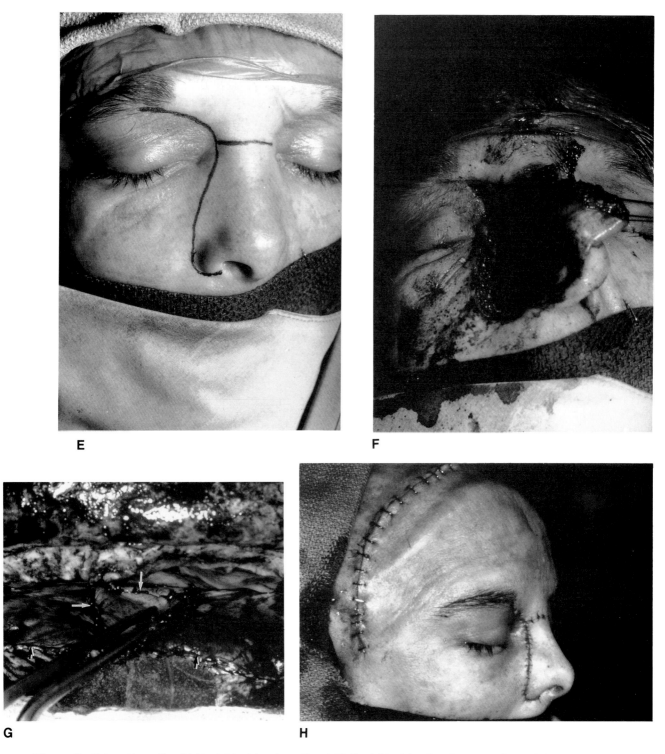

E

F

G

H

Figure 7–9 *(continued).*   **E**: Facial incision is outlined. **F**: Facial incision has been made, and the nose has been retracted toward the left. **G**: Extradural view through the craniotomy flap. Note the closed dural incision (arrowheads). An intradural dissection was necessary because the tumor had invaded, causing a CSF leak. The invaded dura was resected, and a free patch graft utilizing pericranium and fascia was sutured watertight (arrows). **H**: Immediate postoperative appearance. *(Figure Continues.)*

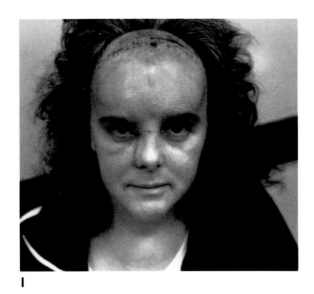

Figure 7–9 *(continued)*. I: Cosmetic result 1 week following surgery.

Likewise, cranial nerves V to XII pass through the temporal bone, and hearing and balance end organs are housed here as well.

A new era of lateral skull base surgery began when John Lewis[28,29] published his series of temporal bone resections for extensive malignancies. The early morbidity and mortality improved, but total bone resection still remains a great technical challenge, with local and distant tumor spread. House[30] added new transtemporal bone techniques for acoustic tumors, as did Fisch and Pillsbury[31] for glomus tumors.

The neoplasms most frequently encountered intracranially are meningiomas, acoustic neuromas, and glomus jugulare tumors and, extracranially, squamous cell carcinoma and salivary gland tumors.

Malignancies involving the lateral skull base, including the infratemporal fossa, pterygomaxillary fossa, and parapharyngeal space, are commonly associated with severe pain. Anything short of complete removal leads to over an 80% local recurrence rate. However, extensive tumor intracranially or into the sphenoid sinus, foramen lacerum, and vertebral bodies may make resection impossible.[32]

For anteriorly placed infratemporal lesions, the approach is similar to the lateral anterior skull base approach. Cranial nerves V, VII, and IX to XII need identification and protection unless compromised by tumor. The internal carotid artery is followed through the skull base and mobilized to facilitate tumor removal. If trapped by tumor, it may need to be resected and a bypass graft placed.

Extensive preoperative evaluation of the arterial and venous circulation is required to assess the involvement and dominance of the vessels. It must be established before surgery whether these structures can be resected if necessary, with or without reconstruction.

If the IX and X nerves are involved, a tracheostomy and feeding tube may be needed to minimize the risk of severe postoperative complications.

In lateral approaches through the temporal bone, the facial nerve is mobilized extensively. Although it may be possible to leave it in its canal, often it must be translocated. Such manipulations frequently give rise afterward to significant palsy and synkinesis as the nerve regenerates. Protection of the ipsilateral eye during this period is crucial.

For neoplasms involving the clivus, sphenoidal area, petrous apex, orbit, middle fossa, infratemporal fossa, and the retro and parapharyngeal areas, a combined subtemporal and preauricular infratemporal fossa approach offers the greatest exposure.[33] If tumor is intradural as well as extradural, staged surgery is planned. A lumbar drain is used in addition to mannitol for brain relaxation. The exposure begins with a skin flap, including the frontal scalp, continuing around beneath the exterior auditory canal and extending along an anterior cervical crease (Fig. 7–10). The internal carotid artery (ICA) and external carotid artery as well as the VII, IX, X, XI, and XII nerves in the neck are exposed and dissected to the skull base (Fig. 7–11). The mandibular condyle and glenoid fossa are removed with the zygoma and frontotemporal bone flap, allowing excellent exposure of the infratemporal dura and skull base. Depending on the pathologic condition, the bone can be drilled away, revealing the entire intrapetrous carotid, the branches of V, the cavernous sinus, the superior orbital fissure, the optic canal, and the clivus (Fig. 7–10). The pterygopalantine and infratemporal fossae are thus opened. The clivus can be removed from the petrous apex to the foramen magnum. For extensive clival lesions, it is advantageous to combine the lateral approach with an anterior one.

Figure 7–10. **A**: Drawing depicting the incision used for the preauricular infratemporal approach to lateral and posterior cranial base tumors. **B**: The skin flap has been reflected anteriorly. A neck dissection is carried out to identify the internal and external carotid arteries, the jugular vein, and the IX, X, XI, and XII nerves. The VII nerve is identified from the stylomastoid foramen into the parotid gland. *(Figure Continues.)*

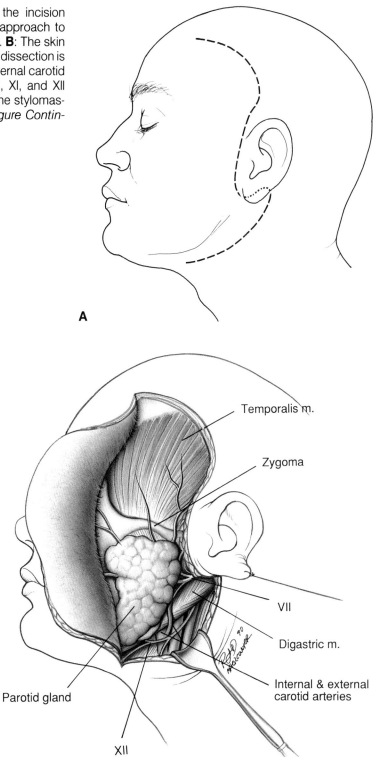

A

Temporalis m.

Zygoma

VII

Digastric m.

Internal & external carotid arteries

Parotid gland

B   XII

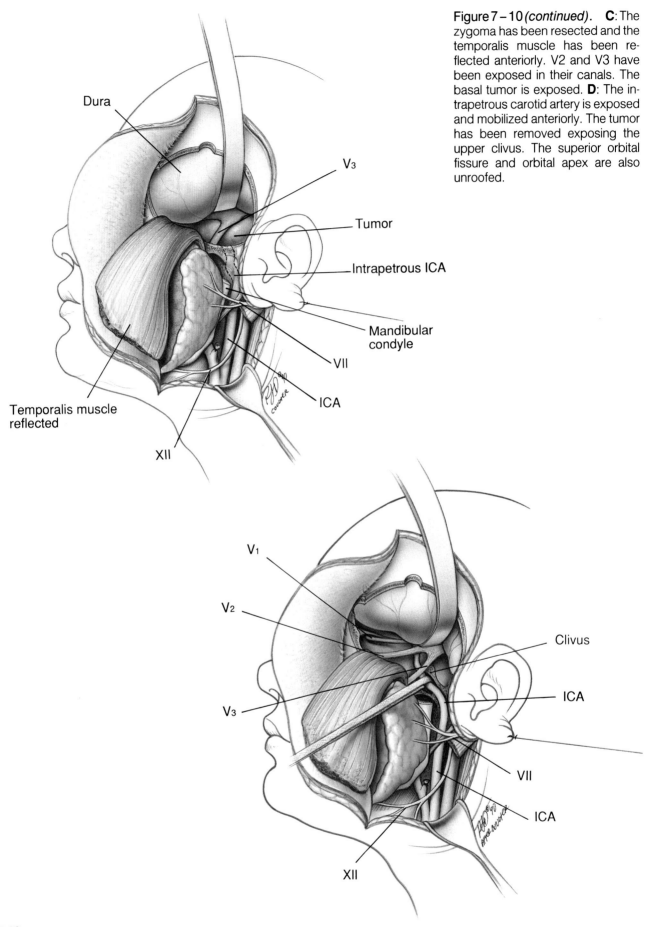

Figure 7–10 *(continued)*. **C**: The zygoma has been resected and the temporalis muscle has been reflected anteriorly. V2 and V3 have been exposed in their canals. The basal tumor is exposed. **D**: The intrapetrous carotid artery is exposed and mobilized anteriorly. The tumor has been removed exposing the upper clivus. The superior orbital fissure and orbital apex are also unroofed.

Dura

V₃

Tumor

Intrapetrous ICA

Mandibular condyle

VII

Temporalis muscle reflected

ICA

XII

V₁

V₂

V₃

Clivus

ICA

VII

ICA

XII

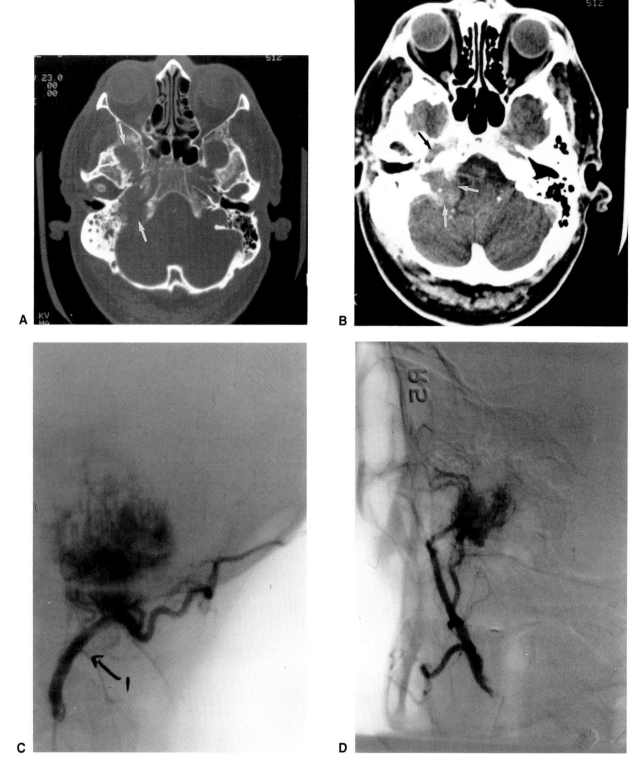

Figure 7–11.   **A**: A 66-year-old man presented 20 years previously with right-sided hearing loss. At that time, evaluation and biopsy showed a glomus jugulare tumor. It was treated with radiation therapy. He now presents with right occipital pain, facial weakness, marked incoordination, and gait disturbance. CT scan with bone algorithm demonstrates erosion of the right skull base from the carotid canal to the jugular fossa (arrows). **B**: Enhanced axial CT scan demonstrates tumor entering the dura in the posterior fossa and extending anteriorly to the carotid canal (arrows). **C**: Arteriogram with selective injection of the occipital branch of the external carotid artery. A large tumor blush is seen. This vessel was embolized. **D**: Arteriogram with selective injection of the ascending pharyngeal branch of the external carotid artery. A tumor blush is evident. This vessel was embolized. *(Figure Continues.)*

143

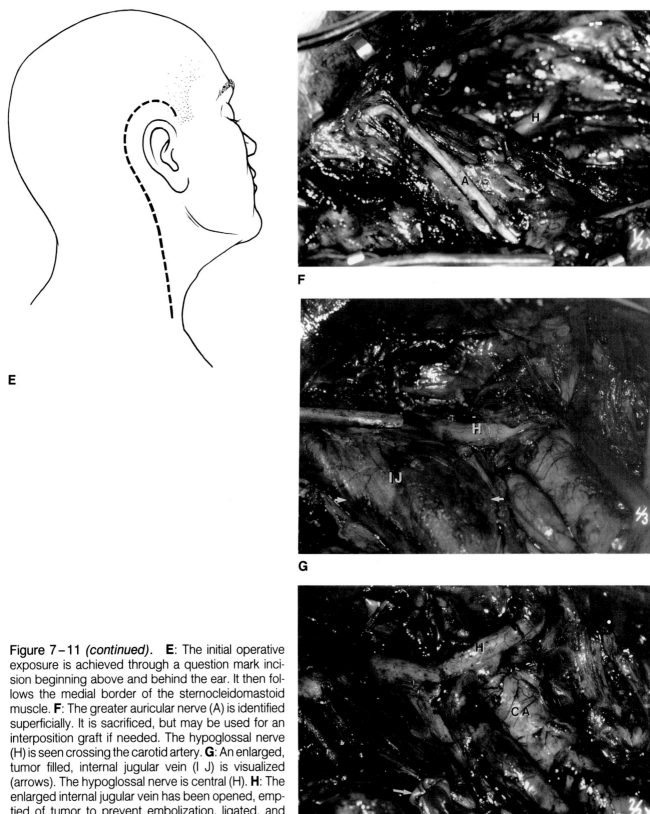

E

F

G

H

Figure 7–11 *(continued)*.   **E**: The initial operative exposure is achieved through a question mark incision beginning above and behind the ear. It then follows the medial border of the sternocleidomastoid muscle. **F**: The greater auricular nerve (A) is identified superficially. It is sacrificed, but may be used for an interposition graft if needed. The hypoglossal nerve (H) is seen crossing the carotid artery. **G**: An enlarged, tumor filled, internal jugular vein (I J) is visualized (arrows). The hypoglossal nerve is central (H). **H**: The enlarged internal jugular vein has been opened, emptied of tumor to prevent embolization, ligated, and transsected (arrow). The carotid artery is well visualized (CA). *(Figure Continues.)*

Figure 7–11 *(continued)*. **I**: The sternocleidomastoid and the digastric muscles have been detached from the mastoid. The hypoglossal nerve (H) can be seen close to the skull base. **J**: The IX(9), X(10), IX(11), and XII(H) nerves can be seen entering the skull base. The tumor (T) is in the left lower corner, somewhat separated from the nerves. A vessel loop is seen about the internal carotid artery (IC). **K**: The tumor is now central (arrows). It has been separated from the lower cranial nerves, which are seen to the right as they enter the skull base. A suboccipital craniectomy has been done uncovering the tumor. The sigmoid sinus was opened and plugged proximally, as was the inferior petrosal sinus anteriorly. The tumor now only needs dissection from the carotid canal, which will be done inferiorly following the artery through the base.

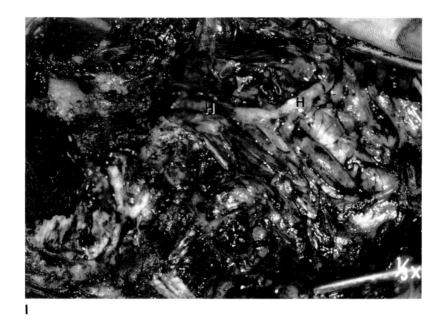

I

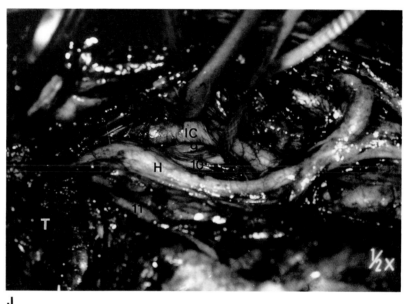

J

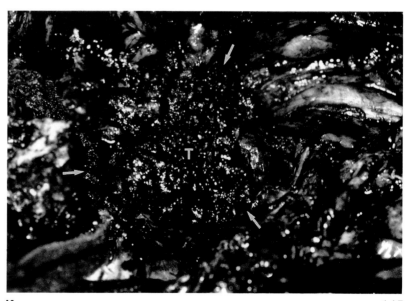

K

The need for maintenance of the ICA or bypass can be determined by preoperative balloon testing, as previously described.

Reconstruction is of major importance. Dural defects are repaired using autologous temporalis fascia, fascia lata, or pericranium. Vascularized tissue is used to cover the dura, especially if it communicates with the nasopharynx or paranasal sinuses. Temporalis muscle or a vascularized graft from the latissimus dorsi, trapezius, or rectus abdominis muscle is utilized and separates the dura from the structures below. Skin grafts are not necessary in the nasopharynx, since mucosa grows rapidly.

Postoperatively, spinal drainage is maintained for 3 to 5 days. Tracheostomy is usually necessary, as is a temporary feeding tube. If there is transient IX and X nerve dysfunction, the vocal cord is injected with Gelfoam or Teflon.

Glomus jugulare tumors are almost always approached surgically, often preceded by embolization following angiography (Fig. 7–11A–D).[34,35] Radiation therapy is considered for poor surgical risk patients, incomplete removals, or local recurrences.[36]

For these inferiorly based tumors involving the temporal bone with neck extension, a lateral skull base approach is utilized (Fig. 7–11). The external and internal carotid arteries are isolated along with the jugular vein and distal portions of cranial nerves VII, IX to XII (Fig. 7–11E–K).

However, in a review[37] of 17 patients with large glomus jugulare tumors, it was found that all 17 had new cranial nerve deficits or progression of preexisting palsy following surgery. The facial nerve was the one most commonly involved, followed by the vagus, glossopharyngeal and, least often, the hypoglossal.

Posterior Cranial Base

A variety of skull base tumors occur in the posterior fossa. The most frequent are acoustic neuroma and meningioma in the cerebellopontine angle.

The surgical approaches employed for acoustic neuroma include a retromastoid, suboccipital procedure with transporus removal of the intracanalicular portion of the lesion for all sizes of tumors, a translabyrinthine approach for small or medium-sized tumors, and a middle fossa approach for intracanalicular tumors. The choice of specific approach depends on multiple factors, such as tumor size, status of preoperative hearing, and preference of the surgeon. Hearing cannot be spared with a translabyrinthine operation.

The use of microsurgical techniques and sophisticated monitoring for brainstem auditory evoked responses and VII nerve function should produce excellent results. Nevertheless, with large tumors, the VII, IX, and X nerves may be functionally, if not anatomically, lost.

Tumors of the clivus are most often chordomas or meningiomas. Both may require combined surgical procedures, including an intradural posterior fossa resection, along with an anterior skull base or lateral skull base approach. As we become more experienced with basal skull approaches, surgery becomes more successful in reaching these lesions, allowing extirpation and long-term survival.

References

1. Ketcham AS, Wilkins RH, VanBuren JM, Smith RR. A combined intracranial facial approach to the paranasal sinuses. Am J Surg 1963;106:698.
2. VanBuren JM, Ommaya AK, Ketcham AS. Ten years experience with radical combined craniofacial resection of the malignant tumors of the paranasal sinuses. J Neurosurg 1968;28:341.
3. Janecka IP, Sekhar LN. Cranial base tumors. In: Myers EN, Suen JY (eds): Cancer of the Head and Neck, 2nd ed. Churchill Livingston, 1989.
4. Sekhar LN, Schramm VL, Jones NF, et al. Operative exposure and management of the petrous and upper cervical internal carotid artery. Neurosurgery 1986;19:967–82.
5. deVries EJ, Sekhar LN, Janecka IP, et al. Elective resection of the internal carotid artery without reconstruction. Laryngoscope 1988;98:960–6.
6. Tarz JJ, Young HF, Lawrence W. Combined craniofacial resection for locally advanced carcinoma of the head and neck. II—Carcinoma of the paranasal sinuses. Am J Surg 1980;140:618–24.
7. Donald PJ. Recent advances in paranasal sinus surgery. Head Neck Surg 1981;4:146.
8. Tessier P. The definitive plastic surgical treatment of the severe facial deformities of the craniofacial dysostoses: Crouzon's and Apert's diseases. Plast Reconstr Surg 1971;48:419.
9. Derome PF. Craniofacial surgery. In: Schmidek HP, Sweet WH (eds). Current Techniques in Operative Neurosurgery. New York: Grune & Stratton, 1971:233.
10. Westbury G, Wilson JSP, Richardson A. Combined

craniofacial resection for malignant disease. Am J Surg 1976;130:463.

11. Sisson GA, Bytell DE, Becker SP. Carcinoma of the paranasal sinuses and craniofacial resection. J Laryngol Otol 1976;90:59.

12. Shah JP, Galicich JH. Craniofacial resection for malignant tumors of ethmoid and anterior skull base. Arch Otol 1977;103:514.

13. Schramm VL, Myers EN, Maroon JC. Anterior skull base surgery for benign and malignant disease. Laryngoscope 1979;89:1077.

14. Shah JP, Galicich JH. Esthesioneuroblastoma — treatment by combined craniofacial resection. NY State J Med 1979;79:84.

15. Chapman P, Carter RL, Clifford P: The diagnosis and surgical management of olfactory neuroblastoma: The role of craniofacial resection. J Laryngol Otol 1981;95:785.

16. Blitzer A, Post KD, Conley J. Craniofacial resection of ossifying fibromas and osteomas of the sinuses. Arch Otolaryngol Head Neck 1989;115:1112–5.

17. Post KD, Blitzer A. Craniofacial resection for anterior skull base tumors. In: Samii M (ed). Surgery of the Sellar Region and Paraspinal Sinuses. Berlin: Springer-Verlag, 1990.

18. Shah JP, Sundaresan N, Galicich J, Strong EW. Craniofacial resection for tumors involving the base of the skull. Am J Surg 1987;154:352–8.

19. Post KD, Stein BM. Technique for spinal drainage: A technical note. Neurosurgery 1979;3:255.

20. Schuller DE, Goodman JH, Miller CA. Reconstruction of skull base. Laryngoscope 1984;94:1359–64.

21. Jones NF, Schramm VL, Sekhar LN. Reconstruction of the cranial base following tumor resection. Br J Plast Surg 1987;40:155–62.

22. Kinney SE, Wood BG. Surgical treatment of skull base malignancy. Otolaryngol Head Neck Surg 1984;92:94–9.

23. Sekhar LN, Moller AR. Operative management of tumors involving the cavernous sinus. J Neurosurg 1986;64:879–89.

24. Sekhar LN, Sen CN, Jho HD, Janecka IP. Surgical treatment of intracavernous neoplasms: A four-year experience. Neurosurgery 1989;24:18–30.

25. Dolenc VV, Kregar T, Ferluga M, Fettich M, Morina A. Treatment of tumors invading the cavernous sinus. In Dolenc VV (ed). The Cavernous Sinus. A Multidisciplinary Approach to Tumors and Vascular lesion. New York: Springer-Verlag, 1987:377–91.

26. Barbaro NM, Gutin PH, Wilson CB, et al. Radiation therapy in the treatment of partially resected meningiomas. Neurosurgery 1987;20:525–8.

27. Deutsch M. Radiation therapy in the treatment of tumors of the cranial base. In Sekhar LN, Schramm VL (eds). Tumors of the Cranial Base: Diagnosis and Treatment. New York: Futura Publishing 1987:163.

28. Lewis JS, Page R. Radical surgery for malignant tumors of the ear. Arch Otolaryngol 1966;83:114–8.

29. Lewis JS. Temporal bone resection. Arch Otolaryngol 1975;101:23–5.

30. House WF. Evolution of transtemporal bone removal of acoustic neuromas. Arch Otolaryngol 1964;80:731–42.

31. Fisch U, Pillsbury HS. Infratemporal fossa approach to lesions in the temporal bone and base of the skull. Arch Otolaryngol 1979;105:99–101.

32. Krespi YP. Lateral skull base surgery for cancer. Laryngoscope 1989;99:514–24.

33. Sekhar LN, Sahramm VL, Jones NF. Subtemporal preauricular infratemporal fossa approach to large lateral posterior cranial base neoplasms. J Neurosurgery 1987;67:488–99.

34. Michelsen J, Hilal S, Sane P, Janecka IP. Glomus jugulare tumors. In: Silverstein H, Norell H (eds). Neurological Surgery of the Ear, vol 2. Birmingham, AL: Aesculapius Publishing, 1979:364.

35. Brackmann DE, Kinney SE, Fu K. Glomus tumor: Diagnosis and management Head Neck Surg 1987;9:306–11.

36. Kim JA, Elkon D, Lim ML, Constable WC. Optimum dose of radiotherapy for chemodectomas of the middle ear. Int J Radiat Oncol Biol Phys 1980;6:815–9.

37. Cece JA, Lawson W, Biller HF, et al. Complications in the management of large glomus jugulare tumors. Laryngoscope 1987;97:152–7.

INDEX